Instruc

LET AUGMENTED REALITY CHANGE HOW YOU READ A BOOK

With your smartphone, iPad or tablet you can use the **Hasmark AR** app to invoke the augmented reality experience to literally read outside the book.

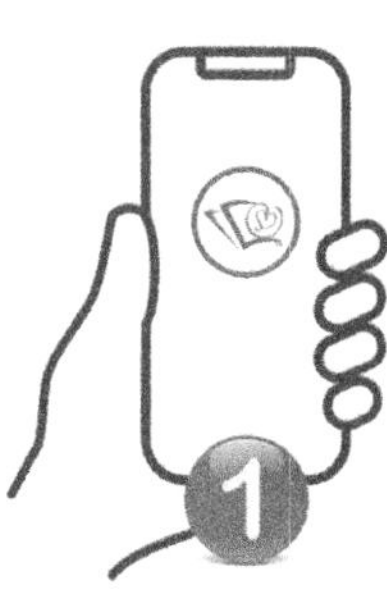

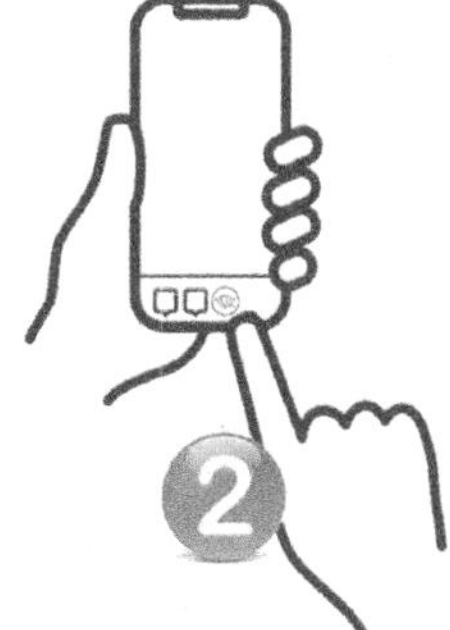

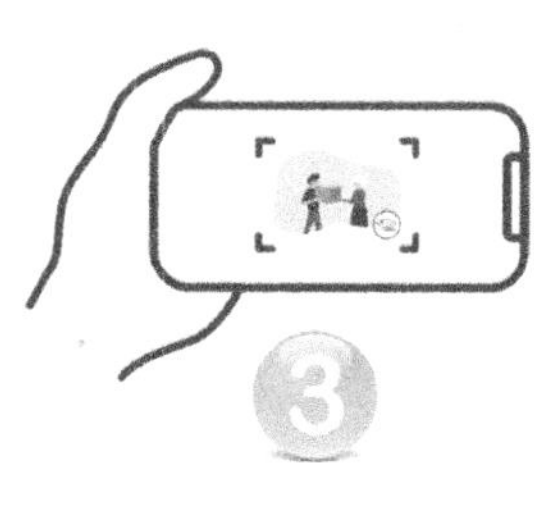

1. Download the **Hasmark app** from the **Apple App Store** or **Google Play**

2. Open and select the (vue) option

3. Point your lens at the full image with the and enjoy the augmented reality experience.

Go ahead and try it right now with the Hasmark Publishing International logo.

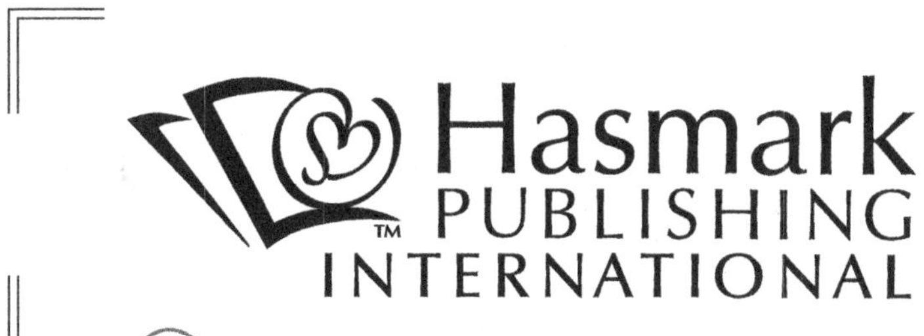

ENDORSEMENTS

Biohacking: Your Way to a Better You' brilliantly redefines aging as an exciting journey of rejuvenation, offering transformative insights for anyone eager to turn back the clock on their health.

~ Peggy McColl,
New York Times Best-Selling Author
http://PeggyMcColl.com

"Dr Grazyna's book is a great summary and philosophy that embraces the power of continuous self-improvement. Her breakthrough discoveries give us tools and ideas for biohacking our journey. Dr Grazyna offers depth of knowledge and understanding into the biohacking that is necessary to develop especially in the world as we now know it. Desire to grow and achieve peak performance, striving for better life and our love to develop our mind and shift the way we think leads us to understand and study ourselves more. Biohacking is not a one-size-fits-all approach. It is a journey of self-discovery and there is so much to learn. This book is truly remarkable, well-referenced explanations and examples make this book an absolute must read if you want to know how to control your health and life. I believe this book is beginning to new discoveries, helping us create our own future."

~Vladimira Kuna,
The Greatest Sales Chic on the Planet and
International Bestselling author of
The Bible of the Masterminds and *In The Realm of the Magic Ruby*

"Dr. Grazyna Pajunen has written her book with great knowledge and compassion sprinkled with authority. There is an abundance of practical steps to take on the road to wellbeing, in an attempt to reverse the aging process. If birth is a beginning and death is our destiny then Grazyna's book is the roadmap. At the end of the day, "Old age is a privilege not offered to everyone".

~ **David Grodski,**
International Bestselling Author of
The Wisdom of Wellness & The Wisdom of Gardening

"I'm pretty savvy when it comes to diet, exercise, the critical role of a good night's sleep, biofeedback, meditation, and stress reduction techniques, but I still learned a great deal of new information by reading (and working on) Biohacking Your Way to a Better You. This book is chock full of well researched, cutting-edge information that will help you to feel better and live longer. After all, what's the point of living a long life if you're riddled with diseases like arthritis, diabetes, Parkinson's, Alzheimer's, etc.? We only want to live a long time if we're going to feel relatively well. Biohacking Your Way to a Better You can teach you how to do that. This is a book that should be studied, not read; readers should put it on the shelf for frequent reference in the future because there is a lot of important, groundbreaking information to absorb."

~ **Sigrid Macdonald,**
Author of Getting Hip and Finding Lisa and
Founder and CEO of Book Magic Editing Company

"'Biohacking Your Way to a Better You' can teach you how to live a long life and to optimize your health throughout the decades. As time passes, we may get older, but we don't have to get sick or die young. This is a book that should be studied, not read; readers should put it on the shelf for frequent reference because there is a lot of important, groundbreaking information to absorb here."

~ **Judy O'Beirn**
President of Hasmark Publishing International

BIOHACKING YOUR WAY TO A BETTER YOU

LOOK AND FEEL BETTER THAN YOU DID 10 YEARS AGO

DR. GRAZYNA PAJUNEN

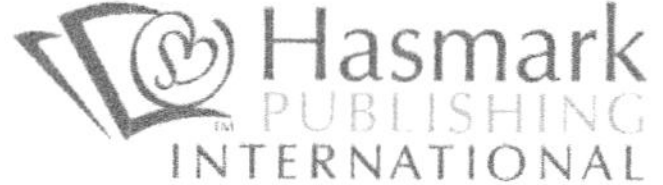

Published by
Hasmark Publishing International
www.hasmarkpublishing.com

Copyright © 2024 Dr. Grazyna Pajunen
First Edition

Disclaimer

Permission should be addressed in writing to Dr. Grazyna Pujunen at gapinvestments@gmail.com.

Editors: Deanna Novak (deanna@thewritejourneys.com)
        Sigrid Macdonald (sigridmac13@hotmail.com)
Cover Design: Anne Karklins (anne@hasmarkpublishing.com)
Interior Layout: Amit Dey (amit@hasmarkpublishing.com)

ISBN 13: 978-1-77482-274-6
ISBN 10: 1-77482-274-1

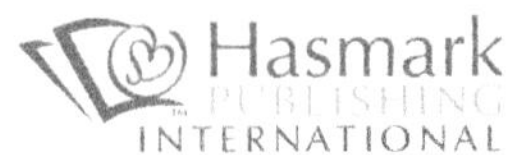

DEDICATION

To my loving husband, Alan, my son Tony, and my dearest parents, who have always supported me in pursuing my dreams. Your unwavering encouragement and belief in me have been my greatest inspiration. I knew that I could always count on you, and this helped me to try and risk more and, because of that, to aim high. This book is dedicated to you with all my love and gratitude.

TABLE OF CONTENTS

INTRODUCTION

UNLOCKING THE AGE-REVERSAL SECRET

In a world where we're constantly bombarded with information about the latest health and wellness trends, biohacking has emerged as a powerful tool for those seeking not just to age gracefully but also to feel and look better than they did a decade ago. Biohacking morphs science, self-experimentation, and self-improvement together. It's the exploration of your body's deepest mysteries—a journey that will empower you to unleash your inner rejuvenator.

Imagine a voyage where you are the alchemist, turning back the clock, reclaiming your youth, and unveiling a version of yourself that's 15 years younger. This is the awe-inspiring world of biohacking—it's a journey that promises to rewrite the script of your life. Each moment is an opportunity for transformation. With biohacking, that opportunity offers not just a chance to age gracefully but to reverse the hands of time.

In the pages ahead, prepare to embark on the extraordinary adventure that is biohacking, where the ordinary becomes extraordinary and where aging is no longer a one-way street. We'll delve into the very core of your being, where we will unravel the miraculous connection between your physical vitality and the elixir of youth. Together, we'll harness the extraordinary power of cutting-edge knowledge to make time itself bend to your will.

Our journey will take us through nutrition and exercise, where you'll discover some of the most basic keys to rewinding the clock within your own body. We'll talk about the importance of sleep, where the fountain of youth flows. And we'll reveal the secrets of hormones, the conductors of the age-reversal orchestra.

But this journey isn't just about you—it's about the world you can transform when you are at your best. We'll investigate both the profound impact of your surroundings on your wellbeing and the moral compass that guides us through the realm of biohacking ethics.

This book is your comprehensive guide to the world of biohacking, offering practical advice, cutting-edge insights, and actionable steps to help you achieve your ultimate goal—a better, healthier, and more vibrant you. It will serve as your roadmap to achieving a better version of yourself, one biohack at a time. By understanding the principles of biohacking and implementing them in your life, you can look and feel better than you did a decade ago and continue to thrive well into the future. It's time to embark on your biohacking journey and unlock your full potential. Welcome to the awe-inspiring world of biohacking. Welcome to the age-reversal secret. The journey begins now.

CHAPTER 1

WHAT IS BIOHACKING?

It's no secret that our lives are increasingly shaped by the rapid pace of technological advancement. But what may be a secret to some is that there exists a remarkable movement—one that harnesses the power of science, data, and human ingenuity to unlock the full potential of our bodies and minds. This movement is known as biohacking, and it is reshaping the way we approach health, wellbeing, and personal transformation.

Defining Biohacking

Biohacking is the art and science of optimizing and improving one's biological functions, physically and mentally, through systematic self-experimentation and the use of cutting-edge knowledge. In this journey of self-discovery, individuals can take an active role in enhancing their health and vitality.

At its core, biohacking is about understanding your body and mind as complex systems that can be fine-tuned for peak performance. To start, imagine your body as a high-performance vehicle and that biohacking is the process of optimizing every component to achieve maximum speed, efficiency, and longevity.

As universal as its benefits are, biohacking is not a one-size-fits-all approach. It's highly personalized, and what works for one person may not work for another. Any journey of self-discovery is similar in this respect because the individual becomes the scientist, the subject, and the experimenter, all rolled into one.

The History of Biohacking

While the term "biohacking" may seem modern, that is likely only because we're so accustomed to hearing about hacking from a technological standpoint. That is not this. This concept with regard to the human body has roots that stretch back through history. From ancient practices like fasting and meditation to the pioneering spirit of Renaissance thinkers, humans have always strived to enhance their physical and mental capabilities.

In recent decades, biohacking has gained momentum as advances in science and technology have made it possible to go even deeper into the intricacies of our biology. In fact, while the biohacking movement is not about technology, per se, it similarly owes much of its development to the Silicon Valley culture, where tech-savvy pioneers began applying principles of experimentation and innovation to the realm of human biology. Today, biohacking is a global phenomenon, with communities of individuals dedicated to pushing the boundaries of what is possible for human health and performance.

The Science Behind Biohacking

Biohacking is a field deeply rooted in human biology. Biohackers are not satisfied with superficial knowledge. Rather, they hunger for a profound understanding of the mechanisms governing our bodies and minds. The foundational scientific concepts that underpin biohacking translate into actionable strategies for personal transformation.

Genetics: Unveiling Your DNA Blueprint

At the heart of your identity is your genetic code. This intricate sequence of DNA molecules carries the instructions for constructing and maintaining your body. This captivates biohackers because it offers insights into our predispositions, strengths, and weaknesses. Advancements in DNA sequencing enable individuals to explore their own genetic makeup, unveiling information about ancestry, health risks, and the potential for optimizing various aspects of their lives. But biohackers don't stop at mere understanding; they use this knowledge to customize their lifestyles. By identifying specific genetic variations, they tailor nutrition, exercise routines, and even sleep patterns to enhance their wellbeing.

One of the most interesting and controversial stories of biohacking from the past involves a biohacker named Josiah Zayner. Zayner gained notoriety in 2017 for his DIY genetic engineering experiment. He was a former NASA scientist who founded a company called The Odin, which aimed to make genetic engineering accessible to the public.[1]

In October 2017, Zayner live-streamed a demonstration of himself using CRISPR-Cas9, a revolutionary gene-editing technology, to modify his own DNA. He injected himself with a gene-editing tool that was intended to increase his muscle mass. This self-experiment attracted a lot of attention and raised significant ethical and safety concerns within the scientific community.[2]

The incident sparked debates about the ethics and safety of DIY biohacking, as well as the potential risks associated with unregulated genetic engineering. Many scientists and bioethicists argued that such

---

[1] Corbyn, Z. (2017). The biohacker who wants to upgrade the human body. Nature. https://www.nature.com/news/the-biohacker-who-wants-to-upgrade-your-body-1.22839
[2] Wetsman, N. (2017). Biohacker Josiah Zayner shows that the human body is a wild ride. The Verge. https://www.theverge.com/2017/10/10/16450616/biohacker-josiah-zayner-crispr-muscle-growth-mutation-ethics

experiments should be conducted in controlled laboratory settings with proper oversight to ensure safety.[3]

While Josiah Zayner's biohacking stunt may have captured the public's imagination and highlighted the potential for individuals to manipulate their own DNA, it also underscored the continuous need for responsible and ethical practices in the field of biohacking and genetic engineering. Serving as a cautionary tale, it spurred discussions about the boundaries of self-experimentation in the realm of biology.

Metabolism: The Energy Factory

Metabolism is the complex network of biochemical processes within our cells that works to transform food into energy and building blocks for growth and repair. Biohackers explore metabolism to fine-tune energy production and utilization in their bodies. They investigate how dietary choices, fasting protocols, and nutritional supplements can influence metabolic rate, fat burning, and overall energy levels.

Understanding metabolism also plays a pivotal role in addressing conditions like obesity and diabetes. By optimizing metabolic pathways, biohackers strive to maintain a healthy weight, reduce inflammation, and extend their lifespan.

Neurobiology: Enhancing Your Brain

The brain is the epicenter of human consciousness and cognition, making neurobiology a central focus of biohacking. Biohackers strive to boost cognitive function, enhance memory, and optimize mental wellbeing. They explore neuroplasticity, the brain's ability to adapt and rewire itself, through practices like meditation, neurofeedback, and nootropic supplements.

---

[3] Mullin, E. (2017). DIY CRISPR kits bring genetic engineering to your kitchen bench. MIT Technology Review. https://www.technologyreview.com/2017/11/27/149877/diy-crispr-kits-bring-genetic-engineering-to-your-kitchen-bench/

Moreover, biohackers lead research into brain-computer interfaces, merging technology with the human brain to augment sensory perception and communication abilities. This holds promise for individuals with disabilities and has the potential to unlock new dimensions of human potential.

Epigenetics: Environmental Influence on Genes

Epigenetics investigates how external factors, such as diet, stress, and environmental toxins, can modify the activity of our genes. Biohackers are keenly interested in epigenetics because it empowers them to control gene expression. By making conscious lifestyle choices, biohackers can positively impact their health and longevity. For instance, certain dietary compounds like resveratrol and sulforaphane can activate genes linked to longevity and disease resistance. By incorporating these compounds into their diets, biohackers optimize their genetic expression for a healthier, longer life.

Cutting-Edge Research: From Lab to Lifestyle

Biohackers aren't passive recipients of scientific knowledge. Rather, they actively engage with the latest research findings. Recent breakthroughs in genetics, metabolism, neurobiology, and epigenetics are now transforming into practical strategies for personal transformation. By staying at the forefront of scientific discovery, biohackers have the potential to redefine the rules of human biology and push the boundaries of what it means to be human. Specific biohacking practices and techniques, each deeply rooted in the profound science introduced in this book, can help you embark on your journey of self-optimization and transformation.

The Philosophical Foundations of Biohacking

By exploring the philosophical underpinnings of biohacking, we can shed light on its core principles that emphasize continuous self-improvement, empowerment, and the relentless pursuit of excellence.

It's important to explore how biohacking aligns with age-old philosophies that have sought to unlock the secrets of human potential.

Continuous Self-Improvement

Biohacking is fundamentally rooted in the concept of continuous self-improvement. It encourages individuals to view themselves as dynamic entities capable of growth and enhancement. This philosophy resonates with the ideas of philosophers like Aristotle, who advocated for the pursuit of excellence as a lifelong endeavor.

Aristotle's "eudaimonia," often translated as "human flourishing," revolves around the idea that true happiness and fulfillment come from realizing one's full potential. Biohackers embrace this notion by actively seeking ways to optimize their physical and mental capabilities. Whether through nutrition, exercise, or cognitive enhancement, the goal is to unlock greater levels of human potential.

Empowerment and Autonomy

Another foundational principle of biohacking is empowerment. Biohackers believe in taking control of their own health and wellbeing, emphasizing personal responsibility for one's body and mind. This philosophy resonates with the writings of existentialist philosophers like Jean-Paul Sartre, who argued for radical freedom and the importance of individual choice.[4] Sartre's concept of "existential authenticity" encourages individuals to take ownership of their lives and make choices that align with their values.[5] Biohackers embody this idea by actively seeking information, experimenting with interventions, and making informed decisions about their health. They reject the idea

---

[4] Donnelly, L. (2019). The philosophy of biohacking: empowerment, responsibility, and radical freedom. Bioethics.net https://www.bioethics.net/2019/11/the-philosophy-of-biohacking-empowerment-responsibility-and-radical-freedom/

[5] Flynn, T. R. (2010, updated 2016). Jean-Paul Sartre (1905–1980). Stanford Encyclopedia of Philosophy. https://plato.stanford.edu/entries/sartre/

of being passive recipients of medical care and instead embrace the autonomy to shape their own destinies.

Pursuit of Excellence

Biohackers are driven by an unwavering pursuit of excellence. They believe that the human body and mind are capable of achieving remarkable feats, and they continually push the boundaries of what is possible. This philosophy aligns with the ancient Greek concept of "arete," often translated as "virtue" or "excellence."

In Greek philosophy, "arete" represents the highest potential of a person, encompassing moral virtue and excellence in all aspects of life.[6] Biohackers cultivate this excellence by optimizing their health, performance, and longevity. They seek to embody the highest ideals of human potential, both physically and mentally.

Biohacking and Ancient Wisdom

While biohacking is a modern movement, its principles resonate with age-old philosophies that have contemplated the nature of human existence and the pursuit of a meaningful life. From the Stoics, who emphasized self-discipline and self-control, to the Eastern philosophies that promote harmony and balance, biohacking draws inspiration from a wide range of philosophical traditions.[7]

In the following chapters, we'll explore how biohacking enthusiasts seamlessly integrate these philosophical insights into their daily lives. We'll see how the pursuit of self-improvement, empowerment, and the relentless search for excellence align with the wisdom of the ages. As we embark on this philosophical journey, we'll uncover the profound connections between biohacking and the timeless quest to unlock the full potential of human experience.

---

[6] Parry, R. (2004, revised 2020). Arete. Internet Encyclopedia of Philosophy. https://iep.utm.edu/arete/

[7] Bellware, K. (2018). Biohacking and the pursuit of self-optimization. HuffPost. https://www.huffpost.com/entry/biohacking-self-optimization_n_5a9a06e5e4b089ec353b7c07

CHAPTER 2

THE MIND-BODY CONNECTION: PRACTICAL STRATEGIES

In the intricate web of human health, the threads of mental and physical wellbeing are impeccably interwoven. Beyond the scientific understanding of this connection, there are practical strategies that can be seamlessly integrated into your daily life to harness this power. In this chapter, we will explore tools that actively shape your mental and physical wellbeing to create unity between your mind and body.

Choosing What You Consume

Consumption is not limited to what we ingest through our mouths. It's also what we consume through all our senses, including what we see and hear.

Limit Exposure to Negative News: The relentless stream of negative news amplifies stress and anxiety and can lead to tangible tension in your body. By reducing your exposure to sensationalized media and opting for balanced reporting, you not only ease your mind but also alleviate the physical burden of chronic stress. For example, I have personally refrained from news consumption for many years, discovering that I haven't missed any crucial information. I prefer to read selected news articles rather than watch television, allowing me to retain control over the content that influences my thinking. During my son's upbringing, we didn't have a TV. Instead, we used a screen and projector to watch chosen programs and movies. This habit has persisted into his adulthood.

Curate Your Social Circle: The company you keep plays a pivotal role in your mental and physical health. Negative and toxic individuals can deplete your mental energy, leading to physical symptoms of stress. In contrast, cultivating relationships with those who uplift and inspire you can nourish both your mind and body. When engaging with someone new, I often inquire about positive events in their life. If they tend to complain, I steer the conversation toward the idea that every situation carries positive and negative aspects. We possess free will and the power to choose our focus. Prioritizing the positive attracts more positivity into our lives, inevitably leading to improvements.

Watch Your Thoughts: Your thoughts have a profound impact on your physical state. Negative thought patterns can create tension in your muscles and turmoil in your mind. Mindfulness practices not only increase your awareness of these patterns but also empower you to release physical and mental stress. By replacing negativity with positive affirmations, you'll observe your body responding with relaxation and vitality.

Harnessing the Power of the Subconscious Mind

Practice Visualization: Visualization exercises engage your conscious and subconscious mind to help you achieve your goals.

One of the most well-documented cases of visualization's impact on athletic performance is the story of Michael Phelps, the legendary American swimmer and the most decorated Olympian of all time. Phelps attributed a significant part of his success to visualization.

Visualization Process: Before each race, Phelps would engage in a detailed visualization process. He would mentally rehearse every aspect of his race, from the moment he stepped onto the pool deck to the final stroke. Phelps would imagine himself swimming with perfect technique, maintaining a strong and steady pace, and ultimately touching the wall in first place. He would also visualize potential challenges, such as turbulent water or strong competitors, and how he would specifically overcome each of them.[8]

Impact: Phelps's dedication to visualization paid off spectacularly during the 2008 Beijing Olympics. In the 200-meter butterfly final, he famously won the gold medal by an incredibly narrow margin, touching the wall just hundredths of a second ahead of his closest competitor. Phelps later revealed that he had visualized this exact scenario countless times in his mind, including the tight finish. His ability to remain calm and execute his race strategy under intense pressure was attributed, in part, to his extensive mental preparation through visualization.

---

[8] Rosner, M. (2008). The Olympian mind of Michael Phelps. Sports Illustrated.

This example highlights how visualization can be a powerful tool for athletes to enhance their mental preparation, build confidence, and improve their performance under high-pressure situations. Michael Phelps's success in the pool, along with his documented use of visualization, serves as an inspiring case study not only in the sports world, but in every scenario and set of circumstances.

Affirmations: Think of affirmations as seeds planted in the fertile soil of your subconscious. By consistently using affirmations related to your health and vitality, you influence your subconscious mind. As your mind embraces these positive beliefs, your body follows with improved physical wellbeing.

Hypnotherapy: Hypnotherapy explores the subconscious mind to address issues like stress, anxiety, and unhealthy habits at their very roots. This aligns the symbiotic relationship between your subconscious and conscious mind, fostering mental and physical wellness.

Stress Reduction for Immune Health

Stress exerts a profound impact on our health, including its ability to weaken our immune system. Chronic stress triggers the release of hormones that can suppress the immune response, rendering us more susceptible to illnesses.

Watch Comedies and Laugh: Laughter, the universal language of mind and body, releases endorphins, reduces stress hormones, and fosters a profound sense of wellbeing. Seek humor through comedy shows, movies, or lighthearted conversations, allowing the healing power of laughter to flow through your mind and body.

Enjoy Every Moment of Your Life: Each moment presents an opportunity for mind and body to harmonize in the celebration of life.

Cultivate a mindset of gratitude, savoring life's small pleasures, and finding beauty in every day. By relishing every moment, you create a type of joy that resonates throughout your entire being. Learn to feel familiar in your joy, positive expectation, and knowing that all is well because this Universe will provide evidence of that wellbeing once you find that place.

Stress Reduction: Stress poses a formidable challenge to the mind–body connection, especially concerning your immune system. Chronic stress can weaken your immune response, making you more vulnerable to illness. Incorporate stress-reduction practices, such as deep breathing exercises, meditation, yoga, Tai Chi, or engaging in hobbies that bring you joy. By managing stress, you not only fortify your mental resilience but also support your immune system.

Stress-Relief Techniques

Stress is a natural and sometimes necessary response that can help enhance performance by providing an extra boost of energy and focus in certain situations. This is often referred to as "eustress" or positive stress.

However, chronic or excessive stress can have detrimental effects on your health and wellbeing. This type of stress, often referred to as "distress," can lead to physical, mental, and emotional problems if not managed effectively.

Effective stress management techniques, such as mindfulness, relaxation exercises, and seeking support from coaches and mental health professionals, can help you cope with and reduce chronic stress while harnessing the benefits of eustress.

Understanding the distinction between positive and negative stress and having strategies to manage stress levels are essential to perform at your best while maintaining your overall health and wellbeing.

Hans Selye was a Hungarian Canadian endocrinologist who is best known for his pioneering work on stress. He is often referred to as the "Father of Stress Research" for his groundbreaking studies on the physiological and psychological responses to stress.[9]

Selye's work on stress began in the 1930s when he conducted experiments with laboratory animals to study the effects of various stressors on their bodies. He observed that regardless of the type of stressor (physical, psychological, or chemical), the animals exhibited a common response, which he called the General Adaptation Syndrome (GAS). The GAS consists of three stages: alarm, resistance, and exhaustion, and it represents the body's response to stress.

Selye's research also led to the concept of the "stress response," which involves the release of hormones such as adrenaline and cortisol to help the body cope with stress. He proposed that prolonged exposure to stress could have detrimental effects on health, and his work laid the foundation for the field of stress physiology and the understanding of how chronic stress can contribute to various diseases.

Hans Selye's work significantly impacted the fields of medicine, psychology, and stress management, and his research continues to influence our understanding of stress and its effects on the human body and mind.[10] In this book, *The Stress of Life*, one of his most famous works, Selye discusses his research on stress and the General Adaptation Syndrome in detail. Selye isn't the only one with these findings. In *Don't Sweat the Small Stuff*, Richard Carlson offers practical strategies and insights for managing everyday stressors, maintaining perspective, and focusing on what truly matters. The book is divided into short, easily digestible chapters, each offering a specific tip or technique for leading a more relaxed and fulfilling life to remind us that there is unnecessary stress when you worry about something you cannot do anything about.

When you feel stressed or overwhelmed, a simple breathing technique can help you quickly release it. Inhale through your nose for

---

[9] Mayor, A., Selye, H. (2017). The stress pioneer. Psychology Today. https://www.psychologytoday.com/us/blog/the-first-idea/201706/hans-selye-the-stress-pioneer
[10] Selye, H. (1956). The stress of life. McGraw-Hill.

8 seconds, hold your breath for 32 seconds, and exhale through your mouth for 16 seconds. Repeat these 3 to 5 times to experience relief.

Additionally, dedicating 20 minutes or more daily to meditation can be highly effective. Quieting your busy mind is essential. To get started, consider using techniques offered by Dr. Joe Dispenza.[11] You can download his meditations and practice them daily to achieve remarkable results. These practices not only reduce stress but also yield positive outcomes in your life and business.

Yoga: Yoga offers a holistic approach to wellbeing, combining physical, mental, and emotional benefits. Through its various poses, deep breathing techniques, and mindfulness practices, yoga enhances flexibility, strength, and balance while reducing stress, improving focus, and promoting relaxation. It fosters better posture, pain relief, and improved sleep quality, making it a valuable addition to your health and wellness routine. Beyond the physical benefits, yoga encourages self-awareness, emotional balance, and self-acceptance, providing a path to overall harmony and vitality. Whether practiced individually or in a supportive community, yoga is a versatile and accessible means to nurture your body and mind.

Tai Chi Gun: Tai Chi Gun, also known as Tai Chi staff or Tai Chi stick, is a traditional Chinese martial art that uses a long wooden staff as a weapon and a tool for physical and mental training. It is an integral part of the broader Tai Chi Chuan (Taijiquan) system, well-known for its slow, flowing movements and focus on balance, coordination, and relaxation.

Tai Chi Gun practice typically includes a series of choreographed movements and forms that help develop strength, flexibility, and awareness. The staff is used to perform various defensive and offensive

---

[11] https://DrJoeDispenza.com.

techniques, and practitioners learn to control and manipulate it with precision and grace.

In addition to its martial applications, Tai Chi Gun is also practiced for its numerous health benefits, including improved posture, better alignment of the body, enhanced circulation, and stress reduction. Like other Tai Chi disciplines, it emphasizes the principles of softness, relaxation, and harmonizing the body's energy, known as "Qi."

HeartMath: HeartMath is a method and technology designed to reduce stress and enhance emotional wellbeing by regulating heart rate variability (HRV). It is a transformative method and technology that places the power of stress reduction and emotional wellbeing into the hands of individuals. By focusing on achieving a state of coherence between the heart and brain, HeartMath offers a unique approach to stress management. This involves using biofeedback tools to measure heart rate variability, enabling real-time awareness of how emotions impact heart rhythm.

Through specific breathing techniques and cultivating positive emotions, you can shift away from stress-inducing states and toward a more harmonious and calming equilibrium. HeartMath reduces stress and enhances mental clarity, concentration, and emotional health. It empowers you to take control of your wellness and find balance in an increasingly fast-paced world.

These practical strategies serve as bridges between the realms of mental and physical wellbeing. They enhance vitality through positivity, mindfulness, and laughter. By reducing stress, you further strengthen the bond between your mind and body, fostering a holistic approach to health that nurtures both aspects of your being while also bolstering your immune system's capacity to protect yourself.

Other Chapter References

Mental and Physical Wellbeing Connection:

1. Chida, Y., & Steptoe, A. (2008). Positive psychological well-being and mortality: A quantitative review of prospective observational studies. Psychosomatic Medicine, 70(7), 741-756.

2. Kiecolt-Glaser, J. K., McGuire, L., Robles, T. F., & Glaser, R. (2002). Emotions, morbidity, and mortality: New perspectives from psychoneuroimmunology. Annual Review of Psychology, 53(1), 83-107.

Visualization and Subconscious Mind:

1. Vernon, D. (2009). Human Potential: Exploring Techniques Used to Enhance Human Performance. Routledge.

2. Dispenza, J. (2007). Evolve Your Brain: The Science of Changing Your Mind. Health Communications, Inc.

Stress Reduction and Immune Health:

1. Segerstrom, S. C., & Miller, G. E. (2004). Psychological stress and the human immune system: A meta-analytic study of 30 years of inquiry. Psychological Bulletin, 130(4), 601-630.

2. Cohen, S., Janicki-Deverts, D., & Miller, G. E. (2007). Psychological stress and disease. JAMA, 298(14), 1685-1687.

Yoga and Tai Chi:

1. Cramer, H., Lauche, R., Langhorst, J., & Dobos, G. (2013). Yoga for depression: A systematic review and meta-analysis of randomized controlled trials. Depression and Anxiety, 30(11), 1068-1083.

2. Taylor-Piliae, R. E., & Coull, B. M. (2012). Community-based Yang-style tai chi is safe and feasible in chronic stroke: A pilot study. Clinical Rehabilitation, 26(2), 121-131.

HeartMath:

1. McCraty, R., Atkinson, M., Tomasino, D., & Bradley, R. T. (2009). The coherent heart: Heart-brain interactions, psycho-physiological coherence, and the emergence of system-wide order. Integral Review, 5(2), 10-115.

2. McCraty, R., Deyhle, A., Childre, D., Theilacker, J. L., & Atkinson, M. (1998). Vagal tone in asthma: Relationships with ecologically valid chronic stressors. Applied Psychophysiology and Biofeedback, 23(1), 1-21.

CHAPTER 3

THE ROLE OF NUTRITION IN BIOHACKING

In the ever-evolving world of biohacking, one fundamental aspect remains the same–nutrition. The ancient Greek philosopher Socrates, often regarded as one of the founders of Western philosophy, recognized the profound connection between our diet and our character. While not a direct quote, his philosophy aligns with the idea that "we are what we eat." Socrates believed that our dietary choices influenced our physical health and mental and moral wellbeing. He emphasized the importance of practicing moderation and wisdom in one's diet, suggesting that a balanced and mindful approach to eating was essential for a virtuous and harmonious life. This perspective from antiquity continues to resonate today, highlighting the enduring significance of our food choices in shaping our overall existence.

What we eat and how we eat it has a profound impact on us, including our cognitive functions and physical performance. This chapter explores the crucial role of nutrition in biohacking, including topics such as fasting and intermittent fasting, personalized nutrition plans, and supplementation for optimal health.

Fasting and Intermittent Fasting

The Power of Fasting

Fasting, a practice as old as humanity itself, has gained significant attention in the world of biohacking. This section examines the benefits of fasting, both for physical health and cognitive function; and specifically, how fasting triggers autophagy, a cellular cleanup process, and its potential role in longevity. Furthermore, the following discusses various fasting protocols and how they can be integrated into a biohacker's lifestyle for maximum benefits.

The Science of Intermittent Fasting

Intermittent fasting (IF) has gained widespread popularity as a biohacking strategy that involves alternating between eating and fasting periods. This dietary approach has captured the attention of researchers and health enthusiasts due to its potential benefits, particularly in metabolism, insulin sensitivity, and weight management.

A. *Metabolic Switch*: Intermittent fasting triggers a metabolic shift within the body. During fasting intervals, insulin levels decline, prompting the body to transition from relying on glucose as its primary energy source to tapping into stored fat reserves. This process, known as lipolysis, not only promotes the breakdown of fat but also contributes to weight loss. A study published in the prestigious journal "Cell Metabolism" in 2017 demonstrated that intermittent fasting enhances fat oxidation, ultimately leading to a reduction in body weight.[12]

B. *Insulin Sensitivity*: One of the hallmark benefits of intermittent fasting is improved insulin sensitivity. A study published in "Obesity" in 2015 revealed significant enhancements in insulin

---

[12] Mattson, M. P., et al. (2017). Meal frequency and timing in health and disease. Cell Metabolism, 25(6), 1256-1267.

2. *Stress:* Chronic stress can affect appetite, food choices, and nutrient absorption. It can lead to overeating or undereating, depending on the individual.

3. *Sleep:* Poor sleep patterns can disrupt hormones that regulate hunger and satiety, potentially leading to changes in dietary preferences and consumption.

4. *Cultural and Social Influences*: Cultural norms and social factors can shape an individual's dietary choices, including food preferences and portion sizes.

An individual's dietary requirements are shaped by genetics, the microbiome, and lifestyle factors. These factors interact and should be considered when making dietary recommendations for optimal health and wellbeing. A personalized approach to nutrition that considers these influences can lead to more effective dietary strategies and improved health outcomes.

Navigating Dietary Approaches

To create a personalized nutrition plan, biohackers need to consider various dietary approaches, including ketogenic, paleolithic, vegan, and others. Each of these dietary approaches has its own set of principles, benefits, and potential drawbacks. By understanding the pros and cons of each, you can make informed decisions about which dietary strategy aligns with your biohacking objectives.

Ketogenic Diet

The ketogenic diet is a high-fat, low-carbohydrate diet designed to induce a state of ketosis, where the body primarily burns fat for fuel. It has gained popularity for its potential health benefits, particularly in weight loss and managing certain medical conditions.

Key Principles of the Keto Diet:

A. *Carbohydrate Restriction*: The cornerstone of the keto diet is limiting carbohydrate intake to a very low level, typically around 5-10% of total daily calories. This is achieved by drastically reducing the consumption of grains, starchy vegetables, fruits, and sugary foods.

B. *High Fat Intake*: Fat is the primary source of calories in the keto diet, accounting for around 70-75% of total daily calories. This includes healthy fats like avocados, nuts, seeds, and oils, as well as saturated fats from animal sources.

C. *Moderate Protein*: Protein intake is moderate, making up approximately 20-25% of daily calories. Sources of protein include meat, poultry, fish, eggs, and plant-based options like tofu and tempeh.

D. *Inducing Ketosis*: By significantly reducing carbohydrates, the body enters a state called ketosis, where it primarily burns fat for energy. Ketosis is marked by the production of ketone bodies in the liver.

Benefits of the Keto Diet:

A. *Weight Loss*: One of the primary reasons people turn to the keto diet is for weight loss. Ketosis can lead to a reduction in appetite, increased fat burning, and potentially faster weight loss, especially in the short term.

B. *Improved Blood Sugar Control*: Some studies suggest that the keto diet can help stabilize blood sugar levels and improve insulin sensitivity, making it beneficial for people with type 2 diabetes or prediabetes.

C. *Epilepsy Management*: The keto diet has a long history of use as a therapeutic treatment for drug-resistant epilepsy, particularly in children. It may reduce the frequency and severity of seizures.

D. *Neurological Conditions*: Emerging research suggests potential benefits of the keto diet in managing neurological conditions like Alzheimer's disease, Parkinson's disease, and some types of brain tumors.

Drawbacks and Considerations:

A. *Nutrient Deficiencies*: Severely restricting carbohydrates can lead to nutrient deficiencies, including fiber, vitamins, and minerals. Careful meal planning and possibly supplementation are required to mitigate these deficiencies.

B. *Keto Flu*: Some individuals experience "keto flu" during the initial adaptation phase, which may include symptoms like fatigue, headache, and irritability. These symptoms usually subside within a few days.

C. *Sustainability:* The keto diet can be challenging to maintain long-term due to its strict carbohydrate restrictions. It may also be socially isolating or inconvenient in certain situations.

D. *Potential Health Risks*: A high intake of saturated fats from animal sources can raise concerns about heart health. It's essential to choose healthy fats, incorporate fiber-rich foods, and monitor cholesterol levels.

E. *Individual Variation*: Not everyone responds to the keto diet in the same way. While some people experience significant benefits, others may not achieve their desired outcomes or may encounter adverse effects.

Below is an example of a ketogenic diet plan for a day:

Breakfast:

- Scrambled eggs cooked in coconut oil with spinach and diced bell peppers.
- A side of avocado slices.

- Black coffee or tea (unsweetened).

Lunch:

- Grilled chicken breast with a generous portion of mixed leafy greens (spinach, kale, arugula) drizzled with olive oil and topped with nuts and seeds (e.g., almonds, sunflower seeds).
- A small serving of sautéed broccoli in olive oil and garlic.

Snack:

- Greek yogurt with a few raspberries or blackberries (be mindful of the carbohydrate content in berries).
- A handful of macadamia nuts or almonds.

Dinner:

- Baked salmon with a lemon-butter sauce.
- A side of steamed asparagus or broccoli.
- A mixed green salad with a high-fat dressing like ranch or Caesar.
- Dessert (optional):
- A small portion of sugar-free dark chocolate.
- Beverages:
- Water with lemon or lime for flavor.
- Herbal tea (unsweetened).
- Sparkling water (unsweetened).

It's essential to track your macronutrient intake to ensure you're within the desired keto ratio, which typically consists of about 70-75% of calories from fat, 20-25% from protein, and only 5-10% from carbohydrates. The exact macronutrient targets may vary based on individual goals and needs.

While the keto diet has gained attention for its potential benefits in weight loss, blood sugar control, and the management of certain medical conditions, it is not suitable for everyone. Its long-term sustainability and potential health risks should be carefully considered by consulting with a healthcare professional or registered dietitian before starting.

Paleolithic Diet (Paleo)

The paleolithic, or paleo, diet is a dietary approach that has garnered attention for its focus on whole, unprocessed foods while excluding grains, dairy, legumes, processed foods, and refined sugars. It has its fair share of benefits and drawbacks, making it a topic of interest and discussion in the nutritional world.

Benefits of the Paleo Diet:

1. Nutrient-Dense Foods: One of the key strengths of the paleo diet is its emphasis on nutrient-dense whole foods. Lean meats, fish, fruits, vegetables, nuts, and seeds form the cornerstone of this diet, providing essential vitamins, minerals, and antioxidants.

2. Improved Blood Sugar Control: By steering clear of refined sugars and processed carbohydrates, the paleo diet can help stabilize blood sugar levels. This aspect can be particularly valuable for individuals with type 2 diabetes or those looking to reduce their risk.

3. Weight Management: Many people find success with weight loss on the paleo diet. Its restriction of high-calorie, low-nutrient processed foods, coupled with an emphasis on protein and fiber-rich foods, can lead to reduced overall calorie intake and increased satiety.

4. Reduced Inflammation: The diet's focus on anti-inflammatory foods, including fatty fish, olive oil, and a colorful array

of fruits and vegetables, has the potential to combat chronic inflammation—a common denominator in various diseases.

5. Gut Health: Some individuals experience improved gut health on the paleo diet, particularly if they have sensitivities to grains and legumes, both of which are excluded from this eating pattern.

Drawbacks of the Paleo Diet:

1. Nutrient Deficiencies: Excluding dairy from the diet can lead to potential deficiencies in calcium and vitamin D. Furthermore, the strict avoidance of grains and legumes may result in lower fiber and certain nutrient intake.

2. Limited Food Choices: The paleo diet's restrictions can pose challenges, especially for vegetarians and vegans. It may also limit options in certain regions, making it difficult to maintain dietary variety.

3. Cost Considerations: Emphasizing lean meats, seafood, and organic produce can strain one's budget. This can make the paleo diet less accessible for individuals with financial constraints.

4. Long-Term Research Gap: While short-term studies show promise, there's a paucity of long-term research on the paleo diet's impact on health. Consequently, it's challenging to assess its safety and effectiveness over extended periods.

5. Social and Practical Challenges: Social gatherings and dining out can be complex while strictly adhering to the paleo diet, given its limitations on food choices. Special requests at restaurants may be necessary.

6. Risk of Overconsumption: Due to its emphasis on meat and fat, some individuals may inadvertently consume excess

calories and saturated fat, potentially leading to weight gain and concerns related to heart health if not carefully managed.

Example of paleo diet:
Breakfast:

- Scrambled eggs cooked in coconut oil with diced vegetables (e.g., bell peppers, onions, spinach).
- Sliced avocado.
- A handful of mixed berries (e.g., strawberries, blueberries, raspberries).

Lunch:

- Grilled chicken breast or salmon.
- A large mixed salad with leafy greens, cherry tomatoes, cucumber, and a vinaigrette dressing made with olive oil and balsamic vinegar.
- A serving of mixed nuts (e.g., almonds, walnuts).

Snack:

- Sliced carrots, celery sticks, and cucumber with guacamole or almond butter.
- A piece of fruit, such as an apple or a handful of grapes.

Dinner:

- Beef or turkey lettuce wraps with minced vegetables and a homemade paleo-friendly sauce (e.g., coconut aminos, garlic, ginger).
- Steamed broccoli or cauliflower.

Dessert (optional):

- A small serving of paleo-friendly desserts, like a coconut and dark chocolate energy bite.

Beverages:

- Water with lemon or lime for flavor.
- Herbal tea (unsweetened).

The paleo diet focuses on whole foods like lean meats, fish, fruits, vegetables, nuts, and seeds while avoiding grains, legumes, dairy, and processed foods. It's essential to choose high-quality, organic, and grass-fed options whenever possible.

The paleo diet offers several potential benefits, including enhanced nutrient intake, improved blood sugar control, and support for weight loss. However, it also presents challenges, such as the risk of nutrient deficiencies and the need for careful long-term planning. Whether the paleo diet is suitable for you depends on your dietary preferences, health objectives, and ability to adapt the diet to meet your nutritional needs. Seeking guidance from a healthcare professional or registered dietitian can help ensure a balanced approach to nutrition.

Vegan Diet

The vegan diet is a plant-based eating pattern that excludes all animal products, including meat, dairy, eggs, and honey. It is rooted in ethical, environmental, and health principles, and it has been gaining popularity for its potential health benefits and positive impact on the environment.

Key Aspects of the Vegan Diet:

A. *Plant-Based Foods*: The vegan diet centers around plant-based foods, such as fruits, vegetables, grains, legumes (beans, lentils, and peas), nuts, seeds, and plant-based alternatives like tofu and tempeh.

B. *Exclusion of Animal Products*: Vegans avoid all animal-derived foods, including meat (beef, poultry, pork), seafood, dairy (milk, cheese, yogurt), eggs, and honey. Additionally, they steer clear of foods containing animal by-products, like gelatin or certain food colorings.

Benefits of the Vegan Diet:

A. Heart Health: A well-planned vegan diet is naturally low in saturated fat and cholesterol, which can reduce the risk of heart disease. High-fiber foods like legumes, whole grains, and fruits and vegetables promote cardiovascular health.

B. Weight Management: Vegan diets are often associated with weight loss and weight management due to their emphasis on lower-calorie, nutrient-dense foods. The abundance of fiber also supports satiety.

C. Lower Risk of Chronic Diseases: A vegan diet has been linked to a decreased risk of chronic diseases, including type 2 diabetes, certain cancers, and hypertension.

D. Positive Environmental Impact: Reducing reliance on animal agriculture can have a positive effect on the environment by decreasing greenhouse gas emissions, conserving water, and reducing deforestation.

E. Animal Welfare: Many people adopt a vegan lifestyle for ethical reasons, as it aligns with the principles of animal rights and reducing animal suffering.

Drawbacks and Considerations:

A. Nutrient Deficiencies: A vegan diet may be deficient in certain nutrients, including vitamin B12, iron, calcium, iodine, omega-3 fatty acids, and vitamin D. Vegans need to pay special attention to ensure they get enough of these nutrients through fortified foods or supplements.

B. Protein Sources: While there are numerous plant-based protein sources, vegans need to vary their protein intake to ensure they get all essential amino acids. Combining different protein-rich foods like legumes, grains, nuts, and seeds can help achieve this.

C. Social and Practical Challenges: Dining out or attending social gatherings may pose challenges for vegans due to limited food options. However, this is becoming less of an issue as veganism becomes more mainstream.

D. Meal Planning: A well-balanced vegan diet requires careful meal planning to ensure adequate nutrient intake. Consulting with a registered dietitian can be valuable in crafting a nutritionally sound vegan meal plan.

Here's an example of a vegan diet plan for a day:

Breakfast:

- Oatmeal topped with fresh berries (e.g., strawberries, blueberries) and sliced bananas.
- A sprinkle of chia seeds and chopped nuts (e.g., almonds, walnuts).
- A glass of almond milk or other plant-based milk.

Lunch:

- Quinoa salad with mixed vegetables (e.g., bell peppers, cherry tomatoes, cucumber, spinach).
- Chickpeas or black beans for added protein.
- Dress with olive oil and lemon juice or a tahini-based dressing.

Snack:

- Sliced apple with peanut butter or almond butter.
- A small handful of raw cashews or trail mix (nuts, seeds, and dried fruit).

Dinner:

- Vegan stir-fry with tofu, tempeh, or seitan, and a variety of colorful vegetables (e.g., broccoli, carrots, bell peppers).
- Serve over brown rice or cauliflower rice.
- Flavor with soy or teriyaki sauce (check for vegan options).

Dessert (optional):

- A vegan-friendly dessert like a piece of dairy-free dark chocolate or a fruit sorbet.

Beverages:

- Water or herbal tea throughout the day.
- A glass of fortified plant-based milk, such as almond or soy milk.

A well-planned vegan diet can provide all the necessary nutrients, including protein, iron, calcium, and vitamin B12. To ensure you meet your nutritional needs, consider incorporating fortified foods (e.g., B12-fortified plant milk) and a variety of plant-based protein sources (e.g., beans, lentils, tofu).

The vegan diet offers several potential health benefits, including improved heart health and a reduced risk of chronic diseases, as well as aligning with environmental and ethical values related to animal welfare and sustainability. However, it's essential for you to be mindful of potential nutrient deficiencies and plan your diets accordingly to ensure they meet your nutritional needs. Consulting with a healthcare professional or registered dietitian can provide guidance and support if you are considering or following a vegan diet.

Mediterranean Diet

The Mediterranean diet is based on the traditional dietary patterns of Mediterranean countries and includes an emphasis on fruits, vegetables, whole grains, olive oil, nuts, and seeds, and moderate consumption of fish, poultry, and dairy.

The Mediterranean diet is a dietary pattern inspired by the traditional eating habits of people in countries bordering the Mediterranean Sea, such as Greece, Italy, and Spain. It has been celebrated for its potential health benefits and is characterized by a focus on whole, minimally processed foods.

Key Principles of the Mediterranean Diet:

A. Emphasis on Plant-Based Foods: The foundation of the Mediterranean diet consists of plant-based foods, including fruits, vegetables, whole grains, legumes (beans, lentils, and peas), nuts, seeds, and olive oil.

B. Moderate Consumption of Animal Products: While animal products are part of the diet, they are consumed in moderation. Lean sources of protein such as fish, poultry, and occasionally red meat are preferred.

C. Healthy Fats: Olive oil is a staple fat in the Mediterranean diet and is used liberally for cooking and dressing salads. Nuts, seeds, and fatty fish like salmon provide additional healthy fats.

D. Dairy and Dairy Alternatives: Dairy products, particularly yogurt and cheese, are included but in reasonable portions. Some individuals may opt for dairy alternatives like almond or soy milk.

E. Herbs and Spices: Mediterranean cuisine is rich in herbs and spices like oregano, basil, garlic, and rosemary, which add flavor without the need for excessive salt.

F. Moderate Wine Consumption: In moderation, red wine is often enjoyed with meals, primarily due to its potential cardiovascular benefits. It's important to note that excessive alcohol consumption should be avoided.

Benefits of the Mediterranean Diet:

A. Heart Health: The Mediterranean diet is associated with a reduced risk of heart disease. The high intake of monounsaturated fats from olive oil, as well as the consumption of omega-3-rich fish and fiber from plant-based foods, supports cardiovascular health.

B. Weight Management: The diet's focus on whole, nutrient-dense foods and healthy fats can help with weight maintenance and even weight loss.

C. Reduced Risk of Chronic Diseases: Studies suggest that the Mediterranean diet may lower the risk of chronic conditions such as type 2 diabetes, certain cancers, and cognitive decline.

D. Antioxidant-Rich: The diet is rich in antioxidants from fruits, vegetables, and olive oil, which may help combat oxidative stress and inflammation.

E. Improved Longevity: Some populations in Mediterranean regions have higher life expectancies, which is partly attributed to their dietary habits.

Drawbacks and Considerations:

A. Adaptability: While the Mediterranean diet is praised for its health benefits, it may not be easy to adopt in cultures with different culinary traditions or limited access to certain ingredients.

B. Alcohol Consumption: While moderate wine consumption is associated with health benefits, it may not be appropriate for individuals with specific health conditions, a history of alcohol abuse, or who prefer to avoid alcohol.

C. Portion Control: It's important to practice portion control, even with healthy foods, to maintain a balanced diet, and avoid overeating.

D. Nutritional Variability: The Mediterranean diet can vary by region, so it's essential to adapt it to local preferences and seasonal availability.

Here's an example of a Mediterranean diet plan for a day:
Breakfast:

- Greek yogurt topped with fresh mixed berries (e.g., strawberries, blueberries).

- A drizzle of honey and a sprinkle of chopped almonds.

- Whole-grain toast with a thin layer of olive oil-based spread.

Lunch:

- Grilled or baked salmon with a lemon and olive oil marinade.

- A side salad with mixed greens, cherry tomatoes, cucumber, red onion, and olives, dressed with extra-virgin olive oil and balsamic vinegar.

- A small serving of quinoa or whole-grain couscous.

Snack:

- Hummus served with carrot and celery sticks.

- A handful of mixed nuts (e.g., almonds, walnuts).

Dinner:

- Grilled or roasted chicken breast seasoned with Mediterranean herbs (e.g., oregano, rosemary).

- A side of sautéed spinach with garlic and a squeeze of lemon.

- A serving of whole-grain pasta with a tomato and vegetable sauce, garnished with fresh basil.

Dessert (optional):

- A small serving of fresh fruit, such as a pear or an orange.

Beverages:

- Water with lemon or cucumber slices for flavor.
- A glass of red wine (optional, in moderation).

The Mediterranean diet emphasizes whole foods, heart-healthy fats (especially olive oil), and a variety of fruits and vegetables. It also includes lean protein sources like fish and poultry. Red meat and sweets are consumed in moderation.

The Mediterranean diet is renowned for its potential to promote heart health, reduce the risk of chronic diseases, and support overall wellbeing. Its emphasis on whole, minimally processed foods and healthy fats makes it a well-rounded and sustainable dietary pattern. As with the other diets, though, it's important to tailor the diet to your preferences and health needs and to consult with a healthcare professional or registered dietitian for personalized guidance.

Supplementation for Optimal Health

Nutrient Gaps in Modern Diets

Despite our best efforts, it can be challenging to obtain all the necessary nutrients from food alone. As such, there are nutrient gaps commonly found in modern diets, which require supplementation, including essential vitamins, minerals, and other bioactive compounds in biohacking.

Several factors contribute to nutrient gaps in modern diets:

A. *Processing and Refining*: Processing strips many foods of their natural nutrients. For example, the refining of grains removes essential vitamins and minerals, leaving behind empty calories.

B. *Soil Depletion*: Modern agricultural practices may deplete soil of essential minerals, leading to nutrient-poor crops.

C. *Dietary Preferences*: Dietary choices, such as vegetarian or vegan diets, can increase the risk of specific nutrient deficiencies, such as vitamin B12 and iron.

D. *Lifestyle Factors*: Busy schedules and on-the-go eating can lead to suboptimal food choices and nutrient imbalances.

The Importance of Supplementation in Biohacking

Supplementation is not a replacement for a healthy diet but rather a complementary strategy to address nutrient gaps and optimize health and performance. Here's why supplementation plays a vital role in the biohacker's toolkit:

A. *Targeted Nutrient Support*: Supplementation allows biohackers to target specific nutrient deficiencies or imbalances. For example, vitamin D supplementation can help individuals living in low-sunlight regions maintain adequate levels.

B. *Bioavailability Enhancement*: Some nutrients are better absorbed when taken as supplements. For instance, curcumin supplements can enhance the bioavailability of turmeric's active compound, aiding in its anti-inflammatory effects.

C. *Convenience and Precision*: Supplements provide a convenient and precise way to ensure consistent intake of essential nutrients, such as omega-3 fatty acids, which are crucial for brain health and inflammation management.

Essential Vitamins and Minerals

Biohackers often focus on specific vitamins and minerals commonly lacking in modern diets. Here are some key examples:

- *Vitamin D:* Vitamin D is vital for bone health, immune function, and mood regulation; deficiency is prevalent, particularly in regions with limited sunlight exposure. Supplementation may be necessary to maintain optimal levels.[20]

- *Omega-3 Fatty Acids:* These essential fats, found in fatty fish and flaxseeds, are critical for brain health and reducing inflammation. Supplementation with high-quality fish oil can help maintain a healthy omega-3 to omega-6 ratio.[21]

  Salmon is considered one of the best dietary sources of omega-3 fatty acids. On average, a 3.5-ounce (100-gram) serving of cooked wild-caught salmon provides approximately:

  o **Total Omega-3 Fatty Acids:** Around 1,000-2,500 milligrams (1-2.5 grams).

  o **EPA (Eicosapentaenoic Acid):** Approximately 500-1,000 milligrams (0.5-1 gram).

  o **DHA (Docosahexaenoic Acid):** Approximately 500-1,000 milligrams (0.5-1 gram).

  Omega-3 fatty acids, particularly EPA and DHA, are beneficial for heart health, brain function, and reducing inflammation. Consuming salmon or other fatty fish regularly can be an excellent way to incorporate these essential fatty acids into your diet. However, it's essential to choose salmon sources that are sustainably harvested to support healthy ecosystems and fish populations.

---

[20] Holick, M. F. (2007). Vitamin D deficiency. New England Journal of Medicine, 357(3), 266-281.
[21] Simopoulos, A. P. (2002). The importance of the ratio of omega-6/omega-3 essential fatty acids. Biomedicine & Pharmacotherapy, 56(8), 365-379.

- *Vitamin B12*: Deficiency in this vitamin, found primarily in animal products, can lead to fatigue and cognitive impairment. Supplementation is essential for vegetarians and vegans.[22]

- *Iron*: Iron is crucial for oxygen transport in the blood. Some individuals, particularly women of childbearing age, may require supplementation to prevent iron-deficiency anemia.[23]

Other Bioactive Compounds

Beyond vitamins and minerals, biohackers also explore the benefits of bioactive compounds found in plants and herbs. These compounds may have antioxidant, anti-inflammatory, or cognitive-enhancing properties. Examples include:

A. *Curcumin*: Derived from turmeric, curcumin is known for its potent anti-inflammatory effects. Supplementation can help individuals harness its full potential.[24]

B. *Resveratrol*: Found in red wine and grapes, resveratrol is touted for its potential anti-aging benefits. Supplements provide a concentrated source for bioavailability.[25]]

Biohackers recognize that optimizing health and performance requires a multifaceted approach, with nutrition playing a central role. While a balanced diet should always form the foundation of one's nutritional strategy, targeted supplementation can help fill the nutrient gaps that exist in modern diets. By identifying specific

---

[22] Hunt, A., & Harrington, D. (2005). Vitamin B12 deficiency. British Medical Journal, 331(7521), 152-153.

[23] Camaschella, C. (2015). Iron-deficiency anemia. New England Journal of Medicine, 372(19), 1832-1843.

[24] Gupta, S. C., Patchva, S., & Aggarwal, B. B. (2013) Therapeutic roles of curcumin: Lessons learned from clinical trials. The AAPS Journal, 15(1), 195-218.

[25] Baur, J. A., & Sinclair, D. A. (2006). Therapeutic potential of resveratrol: The in vivo evidence. Nature Reviews Drug Discovery, 5(6), 493-506.

deficiencies and leveraging supplements, biohackers can fine-tune their nutritional intake to support their biohacking goals effectively.

Beyond Multivitamins

Nootropics, Adaptogens, and Performance Enhancers: Elevating Human Potential with Supplements

The biohacking community, driven by a relentless pursuit of optimizing human performance, has extensively explored a diverse range of supplements. These supplements are used to boost cognitive function, increase energy levels, and enhance physical performance. The world of nootropics is composed of cognitive enhancement, adaptogens for stress management, and performance enhancers like creatine and beta-alanine, each of which has potential benefits and risks associated with them.

Nootropics for Cognitive Enhancement:

Nootropics, also known as cognitive enhancers or smart drugs, are substances that aim to enhance cognitive function, memory, focus, and overall mental clarity. Some prominent nootropics and their potential benefits include:

A. *Modafinil:* A prescription medication primarily used to treat sleep disorders, Modafinil has gained popularity for its wakefulness-promoting effects and cognitive enhancements.[26]

B. *Piracetam:* One of the earliest nootropics, Piracetam is believed to improve memory and cognitive abilities. However, scientific evidence supporting its efficacy remains limited.[27]

---

[26] Darwish, M., Kirby, M., Hellriegel, E., & Robertson, P. (2009). Armodafinil and modafinil have substantially different pharmacokinetic profiles despite having the same terminal half-lives: Analysis of data from three randomized, single-dose, pharmacokinetic studies. Clinical Drug Investigation, 29(9), 613-623.

[27] Gouliaev, A. H., & Senning, A. (1994). Piracetam and other structurally related nootropics. Brain Research Reviews, 19(2), 180-222.

C. *L-Theanine and Caffeine*: This combination, often found in green tea, is known for promoting focus and alertness without the jitteriness associated with caffeine alone.[28]

D. *Bacopa Monnieri*: An herbal nootropic, Bacopa has shown promise in improving memory and reducing anxiety.[29]

Potential Risks of Nootropics:

- The long-term safety of many nootropics is not well-established, and some may have side effects.

- Proper usage and consultation with a healthcare professional are essential before starting any new supplement regimen.

- Nootropics can interact with medications, so individuals on prescription drugs should exercise caution.

Adaptogens for Stress Management:

Adaptogens are natural substances believed to help the body adapt to stress, reduce anxiety, and promote overall wellbeing. Some well-known adaptogens and their stress-reducing properties include:

A. *Ashwagandha*: Ashwagandha is renowned for its potential to lower stress, anxiety, and cortisol levels, leading to a sense of calm and balance.[30]

---

[28] Haskell, C. F., Kennedy, D. O., Milne, A. L., Wesnes, K. A., & Scholey, A. B. (2008). The effects of L-theanine, caffeine and their combination on cognition and mood. Biological Psychology, 77(2), 113-122.

[29] Aguiar, S., & Borowski, T. (2013). Neuropharmacological review of the nootropic herb Bacopa monnieri. Rejuvenation Research, 16(4), 313-326.

[30] Chandrasekhar, K., Kapoor, J., & Anishetty, S. (2012). A prospective, randomized double-blind, placebo-controlled study of safety and efficacy of a high-concentration full-spectrum extract of Ashwagandha root in reducing stress and anxiety in adults. Indian Journal of Psychological Medicine, 34(3), 255-262.

B. *Rhodiola Rosea:* Rhodiola is believed to enhance physical and mental performance during periods of stress and fatigue.[31]

C. *Panax Ginseng*: Ginseng is known for its energy-boosting and stress-reducing properties.[32]

Potential Risks of Adaptogens:

- While generally considered safe, adaptogens may not be suitable for everyone, and side effects can occur.

- The choice of adaptogen and its quality can vary, so selecting reputable brands is important.

- Consultation with a healthcare professional is advisable, especially for individuals with underlying health conditions or those taking medications.

Performance Enhancers:

Performance enhancers strive to improve physical performance and recovery. Two widely recognized performance enhancers are creatine and beta-alanine:

A. *Creatine:* Creatine is well-researched and known for increasing muscle strength and power, enhancing exercise performance, and aiding in muscle recovery.[33]

B. *Beta-Alanine*: Beta-alanine is believed to improve endurance by delaying muscle fatigue during intense exercise.[34]

---

[31] Olsson, E. M., von Schéele, B., & Panossian, A. G. (2009). A randomised, double-blind, placebo-controlled, parallel-group study of the standardised extract SHR-5 of the roots of Rhodiola rosea in the treatment of subjects with stress-related fatigue. Planta Medica, 75(02), 105-112.v

[32] Kim, J. H., & Yi, Y. S. (2013). Ginseng pharmacology: Multiple constituents and multiple actions. Biochemical Pharmacology, 85(7), 873-883.

[33] Kreider, R. B. (2003). Effects of creatine supplementation on performance and training adaptations. Molecular and Cellular Biochemistry, 244(1-2), 89-94.

[34] Harris, R. C., Tallon, M. J., Dunnett, M., Boobis, L., Coakley, J., Kim, H. J., & Wise, J. A. (2006). The absorption of orally supplied beta-alanine and its effect on muscle carnosine synthesis in human vastus lateralis. Amino Acids, 30(3), 279-289.

Potential Risks of Performance Enhancers:

- Creatine and beta-alanine are generally safe when used as directed. However, some individuals may experience minor side effects such as gastrointestinal discomfort.

- Adequate hydration is essential when taking creatine to prevent potential dehydration.

Nootropics, adaptogens, and performance enhancers hold substantial potential for enhancing cognitive function, managing stress, and improving physical performance. To maximize benefits while minimizing risks, you should approach these supplements with caution, conduct thorough research, consult healthcare professionals, adhere to recommended dosages, and closely monitor your responses. Prioritizing safety and individual suitability are paramount when harnessing these biohacking tools to reach personal health and performance goals.

The gut microbiome and biohacking

The intricate relationship between the gut microbiome and biohacking is a fascinating area of study that has gained significant attention in recent years. The gut microbiome refers to the complex community of microorganisms, including bacteria, viruses, fungi, and other microbes, that inhabit the digestive tract. This ecosystem plays a crucial role in various aspects of our wellbeing, including digestion, immunity, mental health, and even performance.

A. *Digestion and Nutrient Absorption*: The gut microbiome plays a central role in digestion and the absorption of nutrients. Gut bacteria break down complex carbohydrates, produce enzymes, and metabolize certain nutrients. By optimizing their gut microbiota, biohackers can enhance their digestive efficiency, leading to better nutrient absorption and utilization, which can be critical for health and energy levels.

B. *Immune System Modulation*: A significant portion of the immune system resides in the gut. A balanced gut microbiome helps regulate immune function, preventing autoimmune diseases and allergies. Biohackers are keen on maintaining a diverse and balanced gut microbiome to bolster their immune response and reduce the risk of illness.

C. *Mental Health and Mood*: The gut-brain connection, often referred to as the "gut-brain axis," demonstrates the bidirectional communication between the gut and the brain. Gut microbiota produce neurotransmitters and chemicals that can influence mood and mental health. Biohackers recognize that optimizing gut health may positively impact their cognitive function, mood stability, and overall wellbeing.

D. *Inflammation Control*: Chronic inflammation is associated with a wide range of health issues, from cardiovascular disease to neurodegenerative disorders. The gut microbiome can either promote or mitigate inflammation in the body. Biohackers work to maintain a gut environment that reduces systemic inflammation, thus promoting better long-term health.

E. *Weight Management and Metabolism*: Emerging research suggests that the composition of the gut microbiome can influence metabolism and weight regulation. Biohackers often experiment with dietary strategies and probiotics to promote a gut environment that supports their weight management goals.

F. *Optimizing Gut Health for Biohackers*: Biohackers employ various strategies to optimize their gut microbiome. These may include personalized dietary plans, the use of prebiotics and probiotics, fecal microbiota transplantation (FMT), and even advanced genetic testing to understand individual microbiome profiles. Continuous monitoring of gut health through tools like gut microbiome sequencing is also a common practice among biohackers.

The relationship between the gut microbiome and biohacking is intriguing, as biohackers recognize that optimizing gut health can profoundly impact various aspects of wellbeing and performance. By employing a range of strategies and interventions, biohackers work to create an optimal gut environment that supports their quest for peak physical and mental performance.

Connective tissue degeneration and biohacking

As we age, the effects of connective tissue degeneration become increasingly pronounced. Connective tissue plays a pivotal role in our bodies, providing essential structural support to various organs and systems. Collagen, a fundamental component of connective tissue, is responsible for maintaining the skin's elasticity and the integrity of tendons, ligaments, and joints. In contrast, hyaluronic acid (HA) contributes to joint lubrication and skin hydration.

One of the most noticeable consequences of connective tissue degeneration is the drying of the skin. Collagen and HA are crucial for preserving skin moisture and suppleness, but with age, collagen production naturally decreases, leading to a loss of skin elasticity and the emergence of wrinkles. Moreover, declining HA levels can result in decreased skin hydration, causing the skin to appear dry and less youthful.

Connective tissue degeneration also exerts a significant impact on joint health. Joints rely on a harmonious balance of collagen and HA to sustain smooth and pain-free movement. As these essential components diminish with age, joints can become less lubricated, contributing to stiffness and discomfort. Conditions such as osteoarthritis are often linked to this age-related deterioration of joint function.

To address these age-related issues and support the body's innate healing processes, you can turn to dietary supplements that provide an absorbable form of collagen and HA matrix. These supplements are thought to help replenish the essential components needed for connective tissue regeneration, allowing the body to rejuvenate itself.

Scientific research regarding the effectiveness of collagen and HA supplements is continually evolving, with some studies indicating positive outcomes, particularly in terms of skin health and joint function. Nonetheless, it's crucial to acknowledge that individual responses to such supplements can vary, and it may take time to observe tangible results. Additionally, a holistic approach that includes appropriate nutrition, a positive mindset, and an exercise routine can complement the use of supplements in maintaining connective tissue health.

For those considering supplementing with collagen and HA, it is highly advisable to seek guidance from healthcare professionals, particularly if you have underlying health conditions or are taking medications. Furthermore, selecting high-quality, reputable products and maintaining patience while expecting results are key considerations when seeking to enhance connective tissue health through supplementation.

Connective tissue degeneration is an inherent part of the aging process, affecting various facets of our wellbeing, including skin health and joint functionality. Supplements containing an absorbable form of collagen and HA matrix aim to support the body in its efforts to rebuild connective tissue, potentially yielding benefits such as improved skin elasticity, hydration, and joint comfort. Nevertheless, the efficacy of these supplements can vary among individuals, underscoring the importance of consulting healthcare professionals and evaluating scientific evidence when exploring these options.

In the quest for self-optimization, nutrition plays a central role in the biohacker's toolkit. Fasting and intermittent fasting offer powerful tools for enhancing metabolic health and longevity. Personalized nutrition plans acknowledge the uniqueness of each individual's biology, guiding them to make dietary choices that align with their goals. Finally, supplementation fills nutrient gaps and provides an edge in cognitive and physical performance.

Other Chapter References

Fasting References

1. Harvie, M. N., & Howell, T. (2016). Could intermittent energy restriction and intermittent fasting reduce rates of cancer in obese, overweight, and normal-weight subjects? A summary of evidence. Advances in Nutrition, 7(4), 690-705.

2. Tinsley, G. M., & La Bounty, P. M. (2015). Effects of intermittent fasting on body composition and clinical health markers in humans. Nutrition Reviews, 73(10), 661-674.

3. Varady, K. A., & Hellerstein, M. K. (2007). Alternate-day fasting and chronic disease prevention: A review of human and animal trials. American Journal of Clinical Nutrition, 86(1), 7-13.

4. Patterson, R. E., & Sears, D. D. (2017). Metabolic effects of intermittent fasting. Annual Review of Nutrition, 37, 371-393.

Nutrition Plan References:

1. Corella, D., & Ordovas, J. M. (2014). Nutrigenomics in cardiovascular medicine. Circulation: Cardiovascular Genetics, 7(1), 3-4.

2. Ferguson, L. R., De Caterina, R., Görman, U., Allayee, H., Kohlmeier, M., Prasad, C., ... & van Ommen, B. (2016). Guide and position of the International Society of Nutrigenetics/Nutrigenomics on personalized nutrition: Part 1—Fields of precision nutrition. Journal of Nutrigenetics and Nutrigenomics, 9(1), 12-27.

Microbiome References:

- Sonnenburg, J. L., & Bäckhed, F. (2016). Diet–microbiota interactions as moderators of human metabolism. Nature, 535(7610), 56-64.

- Lynch, S. V., & Pedersen, O. (2016). The human intestinal microbiome in health and disease. New England Journal of Medicine, 375(24), 2369-2379.

Other References:

- St-Onge, M. P., Mikic, A., & Pietrolungo, C. E. (2016). Effects of diet on sleep quality. Advances in Nutrition, 7(5), 938-949.

- Epel, E. S., Tomiyama, A. J., Mason, A. E., Laraia, B. A., Hartman, W., Ready, K., ... & Daubenmier, J. (2014). The reward-based eating drive scale: a self-report index of reward-based eating. PloS One, 9(6), e101350.

Ketogenic References:

- Paoli, A., Rubini, A., Volek, J. S., & Grimaldi, K. A. (2013). Beyond weight loss: A review of the therapeutic uses of very-low-carbohydrate (ketogenic) diets. European Journal of Clinical Nutrition, 67(8), 789-796.

- Gibson, A. A., Seimon, R. V., Lee, C. M. Y., Ayre, J., Franklin, J., Markovic, T. P., ... & Sainsbury, A. (2015). Do ketogenic diets really suppress appetite? A systematic review and meta-analysis. Obesity Reviews, 16(1), 64-76.

- Gundry, , MD. (2022). Unlocking the Keto Code: The Revolutionary New Science of Keto That Offers More Benefits Without Deprivation. Harper.

Paleo References:

- Manheimer, E. W., van Zuuren, E. J., Fedorowicz, Z., & Pijl, H. (2015). Paleolithic nutrition for metabolic syndrome: Systematic review and meta-analysis. The American Journal of Clinical Nutrition, 102(4), 922-932.

- Genoni, A., Christophersen, C. T., Lo, J., Devine, A., & Bruce, C. R. (2019). The cardiovascular effects of a meat-based diet in people with type 2 diabetes: A randomized crossover study. Cardiovascular Diabetology, 18(1), 1-12.

Vegan References:

- Le, L. T., & Sabaté, J. (2014). Beyond meatless, the health effects of vegan diets: Findings from the Adventist cohorts. Nutrients, 6(6), 2131-2147.

- Dinu, M., Abbate, R., Gensini, G. F., Casini, A., & Sofi, F. (2017). Vegetarian, vegan diets and multiple health outcomes: A systematic review with meta-analysis of observational studies. Critical Reviews in Food Science and Nutrition, 57(17), 3640-3649.

Mediterranean References:

- Estruch, R., Ros, E., Salas-Salvadó, J., Covas, M. I., Corella, D., Arós, F., ... & Lapetra, J. (2018). Primary prevention of cardiovascular disease with a Mediterranean diet supplemented with extra-virgin olive oil or nuts. New England Journal of Medicine, 378(25), e34.

- Sofi, F., Macchi, C., Abbate, R., Gensini, G. F., & Casini, A. (2014). Mediterranean diet and health status: an updated meta-analysis and a proposal for a literature-based adherence score. Public Health Nutrition, 17(12), 2769-2782.

Other References

- Sonnenburg, J. L., & Sonnenburg, E. D. (2019). The Good Gut: Taking Control of Your Weight, Your Mood, and Your Long-Term Health. Penguin Books.

- Mayer, E. A., Knight, R., Mazmanian, S. K., Cryan, J. F., & Tillisch, K. (2014). Gut microbes and the brain: Paradigm shift in neuroscience. Journal of Neuroscience, 34(46), 15490-15496.

- Wu, H. J., & Wu, E. (2012). The role of gut microbiota in immune homeostasis and autoimmunity. Gut Microbes, 3(1), 4-14.

- Turnbaugh, P. J., Ley, R. E., Mahowald, M. A., Magrini, V., Mardis, E. R., & Gordon, J. I. (2006). An obesity-associated gut microbiome with increased capacity for energy harvest. Nature, 444(7122), 1027-1031.

For more information, visit: http://AgeReversingSecret.com

THE IMPORTANCE OF PHYSICAL ACTIVITY, HIIT, STRENGTH TRAINING, AND RECOVERY IN BIOHACKING

The journey toward optimal health, performance, and longevity begins with physical activity and ends with recovery. This chapter explores the pivotal role of staying active, the power of High-Intensity Interval Training (HIIT), the significance of strength training and muscle building, and the art of optimizing recovery through sleep biohacking.

Physical Activity: The Foundation of Biohacking

In an era where sedentary lifestyles have become the norm rather than the exception, the significance of physical activity cannot be overstated. A sedentary existence is associated with numerous health issues, including obesity, cardiovascular diseases, and mental health challenges. Biohackers recognize that physical activity is the cornerstone of their journey, promoting longevity and overall wellbeing.

The Rewards of Regular Exercise

Regular physical activity brings a treasure trove of benefits. It enhances cardiovascular health, elevates mood, sharpens cognitive function, and bolsters metabolic efficiency. When we dive deep into the science behind these advantages, we discover how exercise positively influences metabolism, boosts immune function, and serves as a powerful stress management tool. A comprehensive grasp of these benefits underscores the necessity of integrating physical activity into the biohacker's lifestyle.

Here's a breakdown of the claims with some references:

1. *Reducing the risk of cancer by 40%:* Numerous studies have shown that regular exercise is associated with a reduced risk of certain types of cancer, including breast, colon, and lung cancer. One reference is a review article published in the journal "Cancer Epidemiology, Biomarkers & Prevention" in 2017 titled "Physical Activity and Cancer Risk: Mechanistic Insights." However, the reduction in risk may vary depending on the type of cancer and other factors.

2. *Cutting the risk of stroke by 45%:* Regular physical activity has been linked to a reduced risk of stroke. A study published in the journal "Stroke" in 2013 titled "Physical Activity and Risk of Stroke in Women" found that women who were physically active had a lower risk of stroke. The exact percentage reduction may vary among studies and individuals.

3. *Slashing the risk of diabetes by 50%:* Exercise is known to help improve insulin sensitivity and reduce the risk of type 2 diabetes. A study published in the New England Journal of Medicine in 2001 titled "Reduction in the Incidence of Type

2 Diabetes with Lifestyle Intervention or Metformin" demonstrated the benefits of lifestyle changes, including increased physical activity, in reducing the risk of diabetes. However, the percentage reduction may vary based on factors like the duration and intensity of exercise.

4. *Halving the risk of premature death from heart disease*: Regular exercise is a well-established way to reduce the risk of heart disease. The American Heart Association recommends physical activity for heart health. While it can significantly lower the risk, the exact percentage reduction may vary depending on various factors, including genetics and general health.

5. *Protecting women from osteoporosis*: Weight-bearing exercises, such as walking, running, and resistance training, promote bone health and reduce the risk of osteoporosis. The National Osteoporosis Foundation suggests exercise as part of a comprehensive approach to bone health. However, the degree of protection may vary among individuals.

It's important to remember that these percentages are general estimates and that individual results may differ. Additionally, the specific benefits of exercise depend on the type, duration, and intensity of physical activity, as well as an individual's overall lifestyle and health habits.

High-Intensity Interval Training (HIIT): The Efficient Biohacker's Workout

High-Intensity Interval Training (HIIT) is a popular and effective workout strategy that offers numerous metabolic benefits, fat loss potential, and time-saving virtues. It has emerged as a darling of the biohacking world due to its time-efficient and effective nature. The science behind HIIT involves short bursts of intense exercise followed by brief recovery periods, yielding impressive results. There are various HIIT protocols, such as Tabata, 4x4, and the Wingate method, as well as practical strategies for seamlessly incorporating HIIT into your biohacker's workout regimen.

Metabolic Benefits:

A. *Improved Cardiovascular Health*: HIIT has been shown to improve cardiovascular fitness by increasing VO2 max, lowering blood pressure, and reducing the risk of heart disease.

B. *Enhanced Insulin Sensitivity*: HIIT can improve insulin sensitivity, helping to regulate blood sugar levels and potentially reducing the risk of type 2 diabetes.

C. *Increased Caloric Burn*: HIIT burns more calories in a shorter time than steady-state cardio due to the afterburn effect (excess post-exercise oxygen consumption or EPOC). This means you continue burning calories even after your workout.

D. *Fat Loss*: HIIT is highly effective for fat loss as it targets both subcutaneous and visceral fat, and it can help preserve lean muscle mass.

E. *Time Efficiency:* HIIT workouts are shorter, typically 10 to 30 minutes, making them ideal for individuals with busy schedules.

HIIT Protocols:

A. *Tabata:* The Tabata protocol involves 20 seconds of all-out effort followed by 10 seconds of rest, repeated for 4 minutes (8 cycles). It's excellent for increasing aerobic and anaerobic fitness.

B. *4x4 (or Four-by-Four):* This protocol includes 4 minutes of high-intensity exercise at 90-95% of your maximum heart rate, followed by 3 minutes of active recovery at 70% of your max heart rate. This cycle is repeated 4 times. It's effective for building endurance and improving cardiovascular health.

C. *The Wingate Method:* This is an intense protocol commonly used on stationary bikes. It consists of 30 seconds of all-out effort followed by 4.5 minutes of recovery, repeated for several cycles. The Wingate method is excellent for increasing power and anaerobic capacity.

Incorporating HIIT into Your Workout Regimen:

A. *Frequency:* Start with 2-3 HIIT sessions per week and gradually increase as your fitness level improves.

B. *Variation:* Mix and match different HIIT protocols to prevent boredom and continue challenging your body.

C. *Warm-up and Cool-down*: Always warm up for 5-10 minutes with light cardio and include a cool-down to allow your heart rate to return to normal gradually.

D. *Progressive Overload*: Increase the intensity (e.g., faster sprints, more resistance) as you become fitter to ensure continued results.

E. *Safety First*: Ensure you have proper form and technique to prevent injury. If you have underlying health conditions, consult a healthcare professional before starting HIIT.

F. *Rest and Recovery*: Adequate sleep and recovery are crucial to prevent overtraining and burnout. Listen to your body.

Remember to tailor your HIIT program to your fitness level and consult a fitness professional or healthcare provider before beginning any new exercise routine, especially if you have underlying medical conditions.

Strength Training and Muscle Building: The Path to Enhanced Vitality

Strength training and muscle building form the bedrock of biohacking, contributing to increased metabolism, bone density, and functional fitness. The physiological mechanisms driving muscle growth and strength development are significant considerations that must be remembered despite the common myths around strength training, including the unfounded fear of bulking up, and we must underline its importance for men and women alike.

Physiological Mechanisms of Muscle Growth and Strength Development

The journey toward building strength and muscle begins with understanding the underlying physiological processes. When we engage in resistance training, whether through weights, bodyweight exercises, or resistance bands, our bodies respond in several key ways:

- *Muscle Fiber Hypertrophy*: The cornerstone of muscle growth is the enlargement of individual muscle fibers. Resistance training induces micro-tears in these fibers, triggering a repair and reinforcement process, leading to muscle growth.

- *Neuromuscular Adaptations*: Strength gains aren't solely about muscle size; they also involve improved neuromuscular coordination. As you train, your nervous system becomes more efficient at recruiting motor units, allowing you to generate more force.

- *Hormonal Responses*: Strength training can stimulate the release of hormones like testosterone and growth hormone, which play pivotal roles in muscle growth and repair.

- *Protein Synthesis*: Resistance training sparks protein synthesis, the process by which your body constructs new muscle proteins. This underscores the importance of proper nutrition and adequate protein intake to maximize muscle development.

Debunking Common Myths about Strength Training

Before going further, let's dispel some common myths that often discourage people from embracing strength training:

A. *Myth 1: Strength Training Will Make Women Bulky:* This myth is widespread but largely unfounded. Women typically lack the testosterone levels required for significant muscle hypertrophy. Strength training can help women achieve a lean and toned physique while enhancing their general strength and fitness.

B. *Myth 2: Strength Training Stunts Growth in Adolescents:* There is no scientific evidence to support this claim. When performed with proper technique and under supervision, strength training can be beneficial for adolescents, aiding in physical development and overall health.

C. *Myth 3: Older Adults Can't Benefit from Strength Training:* On the contrary, strength training is essential for older adults. It helps maintain muscle mass, bone density, and functional independence, reducing the risk of falls and fractures.

The Importance of Strength Training for All Genders and Ages

Strength training offers a multitude of benefits that transcend gender and age boundaries:

A. *Increased Metabolism:* Muscle tissue burns more calories at rest than fat. As you build muscle through strength training, you enhance your body's ability to manage weight and improve metabolic health.

B. *Improved Bone Health*: Strength training can increase bone density, reducing the risk of conditions like osteoporosis.

C. *Enhanced Functional Fitness*: Strength gains translate to improved performance in daily activities, making tasks easier and enhancing overall quality of life.

D. *Injury Prevention*: Strengthening muscles and joints is a proactive measure against injuries in sports or daily life.

The Concept of Periodization: A Biohacker's Strategy

It's crucial to adopt a systematic approach to maximize the benefits of strength training. This is where periodization comes into play. Periodization involves structuring your training program into distinct phases, each with a specific focus:

A. *Hypertrophy Phase:* This phase prioritizes moderate weights and higher repetitions to stimulate muscle growth.

B. *Strength Phase:* Transitioning to heavier weights and lower repetitions helps increase maximal strength.

C. *Power Phase:* Incorporating explosive exercises improves speed and power.

D. *Recovery Phase*: Finally, a recovery phase reduces training intensity, allowing your body to recuperate and adapt.

Crafting Effective Strength Training Programs

As you embark on your strength training journey, keep these principles in mind:

A. *Progressive Overload*: Continually challenge your muscles by increasing resistance or intensity to promote growth.

B. *Compound Exercises*: Prioritize compound movements like squats, deadlifts, bench presses, and rows, as they engage multiple muscle groups simultaneously.

C. *Proper Form*: Maintain correct technique to prevent injuries and ensure you effectively target the intended muscles. You should schedule a session with a personal trainer to ensure you do your exercises correctly.

D. *Rest and Recovery*: Adequate rest between workouts and sufficient sleep are critical for optimal recovery and performance.

By embracing these principles, you'll unlock the full potential of strength training, fostering muscle growth, improving strength, and optimizing your overall health and wellbeing.

Suggested Exercises for Arthritis

Exercise can also be extremely beneficial for people with arthritis as it helps improve joint mobility, strengthen muscles around the affected joints, reduce pain, and enhance overall physical function. However, it's crucial to choose exercises that are gentle on the joints and appropriate for your specific condition. Always consult a healthcare provider or physical therapist before starting a new exercise program for arthritis.

Here are some suggested exercises for arthritis:

A. *Range of Motion (ROM) Exercises:*
   o These exercises aim to maintain or improve joint flexibility and reduce stiffness. They involve gently moving the affected joint through its full range of motion.

   o Examples include wrist circles, ankle circles, and neck rotations.

B. *Strengthening Exercises:*
   o Strengthening exercises help improve muscle strength around the affected joint, providing better support and stability.

o Low-impact options like leg lifts, seated leg extensions, and wall push-ups can be effective.

C. *Aerobic Exercises*:

o Low-impact aerobic exercises, such as walking, swimming, and cycling, can help improve cardiovascular fitness without putting excessive stress on the joints.

o Water aerobics is an excellent choice as the buoyancy of water reduces joint impact.

D. *Tai Chi*:

o Tai Chi is a low-impact, slow-motion exercise that incorporates gentle flowing movements and deep breathing. It has been shown to improve balance, flexibility, and overall physical function in people with arthritis.

E. *Yoga:*

o Yoga can help improve joint flexibility, balance, and muscle strength. Gentle classes or modifications to traditional poses can make yoga accessible to people with arthritis.

F. *Pilates:*

o Pilates focuses on core strength, flexibility, and balance. It can be adapted to accommodate joint limitations, making it a suitable exercise option for arthritis.

G. *Resistance Band Exercises*:

o Resistance bands provide a low-impact way to strengthen muscles. They can be used for upper and lower body exercises, such as leg lifts, bicep curls, and shoulder presses.

H. *Cycling:*

   o Stationary or outdoor cycling can be an excellent option for people with arthritis, as it is gentle on the joints and provides a good cardiovascular workout.

I. *Gentle Stretching*:

   o Stretching exercises can help improve flexibility and reduce muscle tension. Consider gentle stretching routines for the entire body, paying special attention to the affected joints. Yin-yoga will be great for that.

J. *Hand Exercises*:

   o For those with hand arthritis, hand exercises using therapeutic putty or stress balls can help maintain dexterity and strength.

Remember these general tips when exercising with arthritis:

- Start slowly and progress gradually to avoid overexertion.
- Use proper form and technique to prevent injury.
- Listen to your body, and if you experience pain or discomfort, stop or modify the exercise.
- Apply heat or cold therapy before or after exercise to alleviate pain and stiffness.
- Consider working with a physical therapist or exercise specialist who can create a tailored exercise program for your specific needs.

It's important to customize your exercise routine based on the type and severity of your arthritis, so consult with a healthcare provider or physical therapist to create a plan that is safe and effective for you.

Recovery and Sleep Biohacking: The Nighttime Optimization

One of the most powerful and yet often underestimated tools at our disposal in the world of biohacking is sleep. Sleep is a cornerstone of health and performance, and understanding how to optimize it with practical tips and techniques for creating a sleep-conducive environment, managing stress, and harnessing the potential of sleep-tracking technology can propel us further along our biohacking journey. At the cutting-edge of sleep science, we can apply the latest insights to enhance our sleep quality and overall wellbeing.

Creating a Sleep-Conducive Environment:

The foundation of a good night's sleep lies in your sleep environment. Here are some practical steps you can take:

A. *Darkness*: Transform your bedroom into a sanctuary of darkness. Use blackout curtains, eliminate LED lights, and consider wearing an eye mask if necessary. Darkness encourages the production of melatonin, the hormone that regulates sleep.

B. *Temperature*: Keep your sleep space comfortably cool, ideally within the range of 60-67°F (15-19°C). A cooler room temperature is generally more conducive to sleep.

C. *Comfortable Bedding*: Invest in a comfortable mattress and bedding that cater to your preferences, whether you favor a firm or soft sleeping surface.

D. *Quietude:* Minimize noise disruptions with the help of earplugs, white noise machines, or soothing sounds like ocean waves or rainfall.

E. *Limit Screen Time:* Steer clear of screens (phones, tablets, TVs) at least an hour before bedtime. The blue light emitted from screens can disrupt your sleep-wake cycle.

F. *Bedtime Routine*: Establish a calming pre-sleep routine. Activities like reading, gentle stretching, or a warm bath can signal to your body that it's time to wind down.

Managing Stress:

Stress is one of the chief adversaries of restful sleep. Here are some strategies to manage it effectively:

A. *Mindfulness Meditation*: Practice mindfulness or meditation techniques to reduce stress and anxiety. These practices can help quiet your mind and prepare it for rest.

B. *Progressive Muscle Relaxation*: Engage in progressive muscle relaxation exercises to release physical tension before bedtime.

C. *Breathing Exercises*: Embrace deep, slow breathing exercises, which activate your parasympathetic nervous system, promoting relaxation. Try techniques like the 4-7-8 or 8-32-16 or diaphragmatic breathing.

D. *Caffeine and Alcohol*: Steer clear of caffeine and alcohol in the hours leading up to bedtime, as they can disrupt your sleep patterns.

E. *Journaling:* Jot down your thoughts and concerns in a journal before retiring for the night. This simple practice can help clear your mind.

Harnessing Sleep-Tracking Technology:

Technology can be a powerful ally in your quest for optimal sleep. Here's how to make the most of it:

A. *Wearable Devices*: Consider utilizing wearable fitness trackers or smartwatches that monitor your sleep patterns. These devices can offer valuable insights into the duration and quality of your sleep.

B. *Smartphone Apps*: Numerous sleep-tracking apps are available that use your smartphone's accelerometer to analyze your sleep patterns. Some even provide personalized sleep improvement recommendations.

C. *Sleep Monitors*: For a more comprehensive analysis, invest in dedicated sleep monitoring devices that offer in-depth data.

D. *Data Interpretation*: Leverage the data collected by these devices to identify trends and patterns in your sleep. Use this information to fine-tune your sleep schedule, bedtime routine, and sleep environment.

Cutting-Edge Sleep Science:

To stay ahead in your biohacking journey, stay informed about the latest developments in sleep science:

A. *Chronobiology:* Explore the fascinating world of circadian rhythms and their profound impact on sleep and overall health.

B. *Sleep Genetics*: Delve into the emerging field of sleep genetics to understand how your genes influence your sleep patterns and susceptibility to sleep disorders.

C. *Sleep and Brain Health:* Stay abreast of research on the intricate relationship between sleep and cognitive function, memory consolidation, and overall brain health.

D. *Sleep Disorders*: Keep an eye on advances in the diagnosis and treatment of sleep disorders such as sleep apnea and insomnia.

Sleep is a vital pillar of your biohacking journey (we have a whole chapter dedicated to it next), and by optimizing it through a conducive environment, stress management, technology, and the latest scientific insights, you'll unlock untapped potential for your overall wellbeing and performance.

Physical activity and recovery are not optional pursuits in bio-hacking; they are the cornerstones of achieving your health and performance aspirations. Embrace regular exercise, incorporate HIIT and strength training, and optimize sleep quality, for they are the keys to unlocking your full potential.

Other Chapter References For more information and recommended exercises, please watch the following video:

[Link to Video: https://youtu.be/1-3ptuJ2GmE]

Don't forget to check the video description for essential details.

You may also want to consider checking out the excellent book by Scott Hogan titled *Build from Broken: A Science-Based Guide to Healing Painful Joints, Preventing Injuries, and Rebuilding Your Body.*

CHAPTER 5

SLEEP OPTIMIZATION MASTERING THE ART OF QUALITY SLEEP AND OVERCOMING INSOMNIA

Sleep, often underestimated in our fast-paced world, stands as a fundamental pillar of health and wellbeing. This chapter delves into the profound significance of quality sleep, the role of sleep tracking and monitoring, effective strategies for improving sleep, and biohacks for overcoming insomnia.

I once considered sleep a waste of time and even purchased a course on how to reduce my sleep to just 4 hours a day to have more time for other pursuits in life. However, I was unable to implement it successfully for a very good reason—I became so tired that my overall effectiveness plummeted. Now, I understand how unreasonable and unsustainable that goal was.

The Significance of Quality Sleep

The Healing Power of Sleep

Quality sleep is the body's natural restoration process, essential for physical and mental health. This section explores the science of sleep, emphasizing its role in memory consolidation, immune system support, hormone regulation, and overall vitality. We explore the consequences of chronic sleep deprivation, highlighting its links to chronic diseases and cognitive decline.

The Far-Reaching Consequences of Chronic Sleep Deprivation

In the fast-paced world of modern living, sleep often falls by the wayside as we juggle busy schedules and demands. However, the repercussions of chronic sleep deprivation, which occur when we consistently don't get enough sleep over a prolonged period, are far more significant than many might realize. Serious consequences of chronic sleep deprivation exist, including links to chronic diseases and cognitive decline.

The Toll of Chronic Sleep Deprivation:

A. *Heightened Risk of Chronic Diseases*:

     ○ *Cardiovascular Diseases*: Chronic sleep deprivation has been closely associated with an increased risk of conditions such as hypertension (high blood pressure), coronary artery disease, and even stroke.[35]

     ○ *Metabolic Disorders*: The lack of quality sleep can lead to insulin resistance, elevating the risk of developing type 2 diabetes and obesity.[36]

---

[35] Diekelmann, S., & Born, J. (2010). The memory function of sleep. Nature Reviews Neuroscience, 11(2), 114-126.

[36] Walker, M. P. (2008). Cognitive consequences of sleep and sleep loss. Sleep Medicine, 9, S29-S34.

   o *Compromised Immune System*: Sleep deprivation weakens the immune system, rendering individuals more susceptible to infections and illnesses.[37]

B. *Cognitive Impairment*:

   o *Memory Troubles*: Sleep is paramount for memory consolidation, and chronic sleep deprivation can hinder both short-term and long-term memory.[38]

   o *Attention and Concentration Woes*: A lack of sleep results in reduced cognitive performance, manifesting as difficulties in concentration, attention, and effective decision-making.[39]

   o *Mood Disorders*: Chronic sleep deprivation has been associated with an increased risk of mood disorders, including depression and anxiety.[40]

C. *Physical Health Impacts*:

   o *Weight Gain*: Sleep deprivation disrupts the hormones responsible for appetite regulation, leading to overeating and subsequent weight gain.[41]

   o *Heightened Pain Sensitivity*: Lack of quality sleep can lower pain thresholds and intensify the perception of pain, exacerbating chronic pain conditions.[42]

---

[37] Cai, D. J., Mednick, S. A., Harrison, E. M., Kanady, J. C., & Mednick, S. C. (2009). REM, not incubation, improves creativity by priming associative networks. Proceedings of the National Academy of Sciences, 106(25), 10130-10134.

[38] Killgore, W. D. (2010). Effects of sleep deprivation on cognition. Progress in Brain Research, 185, 105-129.

[39] Goldstein, A. N., & Walker, M. P. (2014). The role of sleep in emotional brain function. Annual Review of Clinical Psychology, 10, 679-708.

[40] Alvaro, P. K., Roberts, R. M., & Harris, J. K. (2013). A systematic review assessing bidirectionality between sleep disturbances, anxiety, and depression. Sleep, 36(7), 1059-1068.

[41] Meerlo, P., Sgoifo, A., & Suchecki, D. (2008). Restricted and disrupted sleep: Effects on autonomic function, neuroendocrine stress systems, and stress responsivity. Sleep Medicine Reviews, 12(3), 197-210.

[42] Breslau, N., Roth, T., Rosenthal, L., & Andreski, P. (1996). Sleep disturbance and psychiatric disorders: A longitudinal epidemiological study of young adults. Biological Psychiatry, 39(6), 411-418.

   o *Diminished Libido*: Chronic sleep deprivation may adversely affect libido and sexual function.[43]

D. *Increased Risk of Accidents*:

   o *Impaired Reaction Time*: Fatigue stemming from chronic sleep deprivation can impair reaction times, substantially raising the risk of accidents, particularly in activities requiring sharp attention and quick responses, such as driving.[44]

E. *Mental Health Implications*:

   o *Elevated Risk of Mental Disorders*: Sleep deprivation is closely linked to an increased risk of developing mental health disorders, encompassing mood disorders, anxiety disorders, and, in some cases, even psychosis.[45]

F. *Aging and Cognitive Decline*:

   o *Accelerated Cognitive Aging*: Chronic sleep deprivation has been associated with accelerated cognitive aging and an elevated risk of neurodegenerative diseases like Alzheimer's and Parkinson's disease.[46]

   o *Neurological Consequences*: Lack of quality sleep can lead to structural and functional changes in the brain, impacting cognitive abilities over time.[47]

---

[43] Tarnopolsky, M. A., & MacDougall, J. D. (1988). Sleep, recovery, and performance: The new frontier in high-performance athletics. Physiologist, 31(5), 377-381.

[44] Andersen, M. L., & Tufik, S. (2008). The effects of testosterone on sleep and sleep-disordered breathing in men: Its bidirectional interaction with erectile function. Sleep Medicine Reviews, 12(5), 365-379.

[45] Smith, M. T., & Haythornthwaite, J. A. (2004). How do sleep disturbance and chronic pain inter-relate? Insights from the longitudinal and cognitive-behavioral clinical trials literature. Sleep Medicine Reviews, 8(2), 119-132.

[46] Irwin, M. R. (2019). Sleep and inflammation: partners in sickness and in health. Nature Reviews Immunology, 19(11), 702-715.

[47] Anderson, K. J. (2018). Why sleep matters: the impact of sleep on the brain. The Royal Society. https://royalsocietypublishing.org/doi/10.1098/rstb.2017.0361

Chronic sleep deprivation is a grave concern, as its adverse effects are both widespread and profound. As we navigate our biohacking journeys, it's imperative to recognize the significance of sleep in our overall health and performance. By prioritizing sleep, we can fortify our physical and mental wellbeing, ensuring a solid foundation upon which to build our biohacking aspirations.

Sleep's Influence on Biohacking

For biohackers seeking peak performance and longevity, sleep is consistently a cornerstone of their strategy. Biohackers understand that optimizing sleep is as vital as any other aspect of their journey, and they prioritize it accordingly.

The Power of Quality Sleep in Enhancing Cognitive Function, Mood, and Physical Recovery

In the world of biohacking, sleep is often considered the ultimate performance-enhancing tool. Biohackers understand that optimizing sleep is as vital as any other aspect of their journey. Quality sleep enhances cognitive function, uplifts mood, and accelerates physical recovery, and these insights are firmly grounded in scientific research.

Cognitive Function Enhancement:

A. *Memory Consolidation*: Sleep plays a crucial role in consolidating memories, aiding in the transfer of information from short-term to long-term memory.[48]

B. *Learning and Problem-Solving:* Quality sleep enhances the brain's capacity to learn new information and solve complex problems, improving cognitive performance.[49]

---

[48] Diekelmann, S., & Born, J. (2010). The memory function of sleep. Nature Reviews Neuroscience, 11(2), 114–126.
[49] Walker, M. P. (2008). Cognitive consequences of sleep and sleep loss. Sleep Medicine, 9, S29–S34.

C. *Creativity:* Rapid Eye Movement (REM) sleep, a stage of deep sleep, is associated with enhanced creativity and insight, facilitating innovative thinking.[50]

D. *Decision-Making:* Sleep deprivation impairs decision-making processes, while adequate sleep promotes better judgment and decision-making.[51]

Mood Upliftment:

A. *Emotional Regulation:* Quality sleep is essential for emotional resilience and the ability to regulate mood. Sleep deprivation can lead to heightened emotional reactivity and increased vulnerability to stress.[52]

B. *Reduced Risk of Mood Disorders:* Consistent, restorative sleep is linked to a lower risk of mood disorders such as depression and anxiety.[53]

C. *Stress Reduction:* Adequate sleep helps reduce cortisol levels, the body's primary stress hormone, contributing to a more balanced and calm emotional state.[54]

D. *Enhanced Wellbeing:* Quality sleep contributes to a general sense of wellbeing, leading to a more positive outlook on life.[55]

---

[50] Cai, D. J., Mednick, S. A., Harrison, E. M., Kanady, J. C., & Mednick, S. C. (2009). REM, not incubation, improves creativity by priming associative networks. Proceedings of the National Academy of Sciences, 106(25), 10130-10134.

[51] Killgore, W. D. (2010). Effects of sleep deprivation on cognition. Progress in Brain Research, 185, 105-129.

[52] Goldstein, A. N., & Walker, M. P. (2014). The role of sleep in emotional brain function. Annual Review of Clinical Psychology, 10, 679-708.

[53] Alvaro, P. K., Roberts, R. M., & Harris, J. K. (2013). A systematic review assessing bidirectionality between sleep disturbances, anxiety, and depression. Sleep, 36(7), 1059-1068.

[54] Meerlo, P., Sgoifo, A., & Suchecki, D. (2008). Restricted and disrupted sleep: Effects on autonomic function, neuroendocrine stress systems, and stress responsivity. Sleep Medicine Reviews, 12(3), 197-210.

[55] Breslau, N., Roth, T., Rosenthal, L., & Andreski, P. (1996). Sleep disturbance and psychiatric disorders: A longitudinal epidemiological study of young adults. Biological Psychiatry, 39(6), 411-418.

Physical Recovery Acceleration:

A. *Tissue Repair and Growth*: During deep sleep, the body undergoes critical processes for tissue repair and muscle growth, making it essential for physical recovery after exercise or injury.[56]

B. *Hormone Regulation:* Sleep regulates hormones related to growth, repair, and muscle development, including growth hormone and testosterone.[57]

C. *Pain Management:* Sleep has analgesic properties, reducing the perception of pain and discomfort, thereby expediting the healing process.[58]

D. *Immune System Support*: Quality sleep boosts the immune system, enhancing the body's ability to ward off infections and illnesses, which is vital for a speedy recovery.[59]

Sleep Tracking and Monitoring

The Tools of Sleep Tracking

Modern technology allows us to track and monitor our sleep patterns. Various sleep-tracking devices and apps, with their capabilities and limitations, can be used, but choosing the right tools, whether it's a wearable device, a smartphone app, or a dedicated sleep monitor, is up to the individual.

---

[56] Tarnopolsky, M. A., & MacDougall, J. D. (1988). Sleep, recovery, and performance: The new frontier in high-performance athletics. Physiologist, 31(5), 377-381.

[57] Andersen, M. L., & Tufik, S. (2008). The effects of testosterone on sleep and sleep-disordered breathing in men: Its bidirectional interaction with erectile function. Sleep Medicine Reviews, 12(5), 365-379.

[58] Smith, M. T., & Haythornthwaite, J. A. (2004). How do sleep disturbance and chronic pain inter-relate? Insights from the longitudinal and cognitive-behavioral clinical trials literature. Sleep Medicine Reviews, 8(2), 119-132.

[59] Irwin, M. R. (2019). Sleep and inflammation: Partners in sickness and in health. Nature Reviews Immunology, 19(11), 702-715.

Navigating the World of Sleep-Tracking: Devices, Apps, and Their Limitations

Understanding your sleep patterns is crucial to optimizing your sleep for overall health and biohacking success. Various sleep-tracking devices and apps can help. Armed with knowledge about their capabilities and limitations from the latest research and expert recommendations, you'll be better equipped to choose the right tools to meet your specific sleep-tracking needs.

Wearable Devices:

A. *Fitness Trackers* **(e.g., Fitbit, Garmin, Apple Watch):** These devices often include sleep-tracking features that monitor your movement and heart rate to estimate your sleep stages. They are convenient for continuous, long-term tracking but may lack the precision of dedicated sleep monitors.[60]

B. *Smartwatches:* Many smartwatches come equipped with sleep-tracking functionality. They provide a comprehensive overview of your sleep duration and patterns, including sleep stages. However, their battery life may limit their ability to monitor sleep over extended periods.[61]

Smartphone Apps:

A. *Sleep Cycle*: This popular app tracks your sleep using your smartphone's accelerometer to monitor movements. It provides data on sleep duration and offers features like smart alarms that wake you during your lightest sleep phase.

---

[60] de Zambotti, M., Goldstone, A., Claudatos, S., Colrain, I. M., & Baker, F. C. (2018). A validation study of Fitbit Charge 2™ compared with polysomnography in adults. Chronobiology International, 35(4), 465–476.

[61] Mantua, J., Gravel, N., & Spencer, R. M. (2016). Reliability of sleep measures from four personal health monitoring devices compared to research-based actigraphy and polysomnography. Sensors, 16(5), 646.

B. *Pillow:* Pillow uses your phone's sensors to track sleep patterns, offering insights into sleep quality and snoring detection. It's user-friendly and provides detailed sleep stage information.

Dedicated Sleep Monitors:

A. *Actigraphy Devices:* These wrist-worn devices are highly accurate for sleep tracking. They use accelerometers to detect movement and are often used in clinical sleep studies. However, they can be bulkier and less user-friendly than wearables.[62]

B. *Bed-Based Sensors (e.g., Sleep Number, Eight Sleep):* These devices employ sensors embedded in your mattress to monitor your sleep. They offer detailed information on sleep stages, heart rate, and even temperature control for optimal sleep conditions.

Limitations of Sleep-Tracking Tools:

1. *Accuracy:* Most consumer sleep-tracking devices provide estimates of sleep stages based on movement and heart rate. While they offer valuable insights, their accuracy may not match clinical sleep studies.[63]

2. *Interference:* Wearable devices and some smartphone apps may disrupt your sleep due to discomfort or screen light emission. Dedicated sleep monitors, like bed-based sensors, are less obtrusive.

3. *Battery Life:* Wearable devices and smartwatches need regular charging, potentially limiting their ability to track sleep continuously.

---

[62] Marino, M., Li, Y., Rueschman, M. N., Winkelman, J. W., Ellenbogen, J. M., Solet, J. M., ... & Buxton, O. M. (2013). Measuring sleep: Accuracy, sensitivity, and specificity of wrist actigraphy compared to polysomnography. Sleep, 36(11), 1747-1755.

[63] Montgomery-Downs, H. E., Insana, S. P., & Bond, J. A. (2012). Movement toward a novel activity monitoring device. Sleep and Breathing, 16(3), 913-917.

4. *Cost:* High-quality sleep-tracking devices and dedicated monitors can be expensive, while smartphone apps are often more affordable but may offer fewer features.[64]

5. *Data Interpretation*: Collecting data is one thing, but interpreting it accurately is another. Understanding the significance of sleep metrics requires some knowledge of sleep science.

6. *Privacy Concerns:* Some sleep-tracking apps and devices collect personal data. It's essential to review their privacy policies and ensure your data is protected.

Choosing the right sleep-tracking tool depends on your goals, preferences, and budget. Whether you opt for a wearable device, a smartphone app, or a dedicated sleep monitor, remember that these tools are valuable aids in optimizing your sleep. Still, they may not replace professional evaluation if you have serious sleep concerns.

Interpreting Sleep Data

Once you have collected sleep data, the next step is interpreting it. Understanding sleep metrics, such as sleep duration, sleep cycles, and sleep efficiency, is crucial for identifying sleep disturbances and making informed decisions to enhance sleep quality.

A. *Sleep Duration*: This metric indicates the total amount of time you spend asleep during a night's rest. It typically ranges from 7 to 9 hours for adults. Deviating significantly from this range, either too little or too much, can signal potential sleep issues.

B. *Sleep Cycles*: Sleep is composed of multiple cycles, each consisting of different stages. These cycles include rapid eye

---

[64] Krystal, A. D., Edinger, J. D., & Wohlgemuth, W. K. (2008). Marshaling the evidence on the treatment of insomnia. Journal of General Internal Medicine, 23(8), 1241-1243.

movement (REM) and non-REM stages. Monitoring the distribution of these cycles can help assess the quality of your sleep. A balanced distribution of REM and non-REM sleep is generally considered ideal.

C. *Sleep Efficiency*: Sleep efficiency is a measure of how effectively you use the time you spend in bed. It is calculated by dividing the time spent asleep by the total time spent in bed. A sleep efficiency of 85% or higher is often considered good. A lower sleep efficiency may indicate issues like frequent awakenings or difficulty falling asleep.

Analyzing these sleep metrics allows you to gain valuable insights into your sleep patterns and recognize potential problems. Tracking changes in these metrics over time can help you identify trends and make informed decisions about lifestyle adjustments, sleep hygiene, or seeking professional guidance to improve your overall sleep quality.

Strategies for Better Sleep

Sleep Hygiene

Good sleep starts with a clean slate. We explore the concept of sleep hygiene, encompassing practices like creating a comfortable sleep environment, managing light exposure, and establishing a consistent sleep schedule. These foundational habits set the stage for quality sleep.

The Science of Sleep Hygiene: Building Healthy Sleep Habits

In your biohacking journey, optimizing sleep is a critical pillar of success. One key aspect of this optimization is adhering to the principles of sleep hygiene.

Creating a Comfortable Sleep Environment:

A. *Comfortable Mattress and Bedding*: Investing in a comfortable mattress and bedding that align with your preferences—whether firm or soft—can significantly impact sleep quality.[65]

B. *Ideal Room Temperature*: Maintaining a bedroom temperature between 60-67°F (15-19°C) is generally conducive to sleep comfort.[66]

C. *Darkness:* Eliminating light sources, such as LED displays or streetlights, and using blackout curtains can foster an environment conducive to restful sleep.[67]

D. *Quietude:* Minimizing noise disruptions through earplugs, white noise machines, or calming sounds like ocean waves or rainfall can enhance sleep quality.[68]

E. *Limit Screen Time*: Avoiding screens (phones, tablets, TVs) at least an hour before bedtime helps reduce exposure to blue light, which can interfere with sleep-wake cycles.[69]

Managing Light Exposure:

1. *Morning Sunlight:* Exposure to natural light in the morning helps regulate your circadian rhythm, enhancing alertness during the day and improving sleep at night.[70]

---

[65] Jacobson, B. H., Boolani, A., Dunklee, G., & Shepardson, A. (2008). Effect of prescribed sleep surfaces on back pain and sleep quality in patients diagnosed with low back and shoulder pain. Applied Ergonomics, 42(1), 91-97.

[66] Asplund, R. (1999). Nocturnal temperature and adverse pregnancy outcomes: A review. The Journal of Perinatal & Neonatal Nursing, 13(3), 59-72.

[67] Figueiro, M. G., & Rea, M. S. (2010). Lack of short-wavelength light during the school day delays dim light melatonin onset (DLMO) in middle school students. Neuroendocrinology Letters, 31(1), 92-96.

[68] Basner, M., Samel, A., & Isermann, U. (2006). Aircraft noise effects on sleep: Application of the results of a large polysomnographic field study. Journal of the Acoustical Society of America, 119(5), 2772-2784.

[69] Chang, A. M., Aeschbach, D., Duffy, J. F., & Czeisler, C. A. (2015). Evening use of light-emitting eReaders negatively affects sleep, circadian timing, and next-morning alertness. Proceedings of the National Academy of Sciences, 112(4), 1232-1237.

[70] Rahman, S. A., St. Hilaire, M. A., Lockley, S. W., & Gronfier, C. (2017). The effects of spectral tuning of evening ambient light on melatonin suppression, alertness and sleep. Physiology & Behavior, 177, 221-229.

2. *Evening Dimness*: Reducing artificial light exposure in the evening, especially blue light from screens, helps signal to your body that it's time to wind down.[71]

Establishing a Consistent Sleep Schedule:

1. *Bedtime Routine*: Engaging in a calming pre-sleep routine, such as reading, gentle stretching, or a warm bath, helps prepare your body and mind for rest.[72]

2. *Regular Sleep and Wake Times*: Going to bed and waking up at the same time every day—even on weekends—supports a stable circadian rhythm, enhancing sleep quality.[73]

3. *Avoiding Naps:* Minimizing daytime naps or keeping them short can prevent interference with nighttime sleep.[74]

4. *Limiting Alcohol and Caffeine:* Avoiding alcohol and caffeine in the hours leading up to bedtime can prevent sleep disturbances.[75]

Sleep hygiene practices are essential for creating an environment conducive to restorative sleep. By incorporating these practices into your daily routine, you can optimize your sleep, boost your wellbeing, and enhance your biohacking efforts.

---

[71] Wood, B., Rea, M. S., Plitnick, B., & Figueiro, M. G. (2013). Light level and duration of exposure determine the impact of self-luminous tablets on melatonin suppression. Applied Ergonomics, 44(2), 237-240.

[72] Tsai, L. L., Li, S. P., & Wang, H. J. (2005). The effects of pre-sleep activities on sleep onset in adolescents. The Journal of Adolescent Health, 37(6), 467-472.

[73] Roenneberg, T., Wirz-Justice, A., & Merrow, M. (2003). Life between clocks: Daily temporal patterns of human chronotypes. Journal of Biological Rhythms, 18(1), 80-90.

[74] Lovato, N., Lack, L., & Wright, H. (2016). The energy cost of very short naps. International Journal of Behavioral Medicine, 23(4), 428-432.

[75] Clark, I., & Landolt, H. P. (2017). Coffee, caffeine, and sleep: A systematic review of epidemiological studies and randomized controlled trials. Sleep Medicine Reviews, 31, 70-78.

Relaxation and Stress Management

Stress and anxiety can be major disruptors of sleep. However, there are practical techniques for relaxation and stress reduction, such as meditation, deep breathing exercises, and progressive muscle relaxation.

Unwinding the Mind and Body: Practical Techniques for Relaxation and Stress Reduction

Meditation:

A. *Mindfulness Meditation*: Mindfulness meditation involves paying focused attention to the present moment without judgment. Studies have shown its effectiveness in reducing stress and improving psychological wellbeing.[76]

B. *Transcendental Meditation:* TM is a form of mantra meditation that has been linked to reductions in stress, anxiety, and even cardiovascular risk factors.[77]

C. *Loving-Kindness Meditation*: This meditation practice focuses on generating feelings of compassion and love toward oneself and others. It has been shown to enhance positive emotions and reduce symptoms of depression and anxiety.[78]

Deep Breathing Exercises:

A. *Diaphragmatic Breathing:* Also known as belly breathing, this technique involves slow, deep breaths that engage the

---

[76] Hofmann, S. G., Sawyer, A. T., Witt, A. A., & Oh, D. (2010). The effect of mindfulness-based therapy on anxiety and depression: A meta-analytic review. Journal of Consulting and Clinical Psychology, 78(2), 169-183.

[77] Anderson, J. W., Liu, C., & Kryscio, R. J. (2008). Blood pressure response to transcendental meditation: A meta-analysis. American Journal of Hypertension, 21(3), 310-316.

[78] Fredrickson, B. L., Cohn, M. A., Coffey, K. A., Pek, J., & Finkel, S. M. (2008). Open hearts build lives: Positive emotions, induced through loving-kindness meditation, build consequential personal resources. Journal of Personality and Social Psychology, 95(5), 1045-1062.

diaphragm. It activates the body's relaxation response and can lower stress levels.[79]

B. *4-7-8 Breathing*: This technique involves inhaling for a count of 4, holding the breath for 7, and exhaling for 8. It can help reduce anxiety and promote relaxation.[80]

C. *Box Breathing*: Box breathing involves inhaling, holding, exhaling, and holding the breath for equal counts, typically 4 seconds each. It helps regulate the autonomic nervous system and reduce stress.[81]

Progressive Muscle Relaxation (PMR):

A. *Jacobson's PMR*: PMR is a technique that involves systematically tensing and then relaxing different muscle groups in the body. It can reduce muscle tension, alleviate stress, and improve sleep quality.[82]

B. *Autogenic Training*: Similar to PMR, autogenic training involves self-suggestion and progressive relaxation techniques to reduce stress and promote a state of calm.[83]

---

[79] Ma, X., Yue, Z. Q., Gong, Z. Q., Zhang, H., Duan, N. Y., Shi, Y. T., ... & Li, Y. F. (2017). The effect of diaphragmatic breathing on attention, negative affect and stress in healthy adults. Frontiers in Psychology, 8, 874.

[80] Seppälä, E. M., Nitschke, J. B., Tudorascu, D. L., Hayes, A., Goldstein, M. R., Nguyen, D. T. H., ... & Davidson, R. J. (2014). Breathing based meditation decreases posttraumatic stress disorder symptoms in US military veterans: A randomized controlled longitudinal study. Journal of Traumatic Stress, 27(4), 397-405.

[81] Lin, I. M., Tai, L. Y., Fan, S. Y.. (2014). Breathing through a straw reduces the risk of postoperative atelectasis and length of hospital stay in patients undergoing coronary artery bypass graft surgery: A randomized clinical trial. Chest, 146(5), 1360-1369.

[82] Jacobson, E. (1938). Progressive relaxation: A physiological and clinical investigation of muscular states and their significance in psychology and medical practice. University of Chicago Press.

[83] Luthe, W. (1969). Autogenic therapy: Vol. 2. Methods. Grune & Stratton.

Biohacks for Overcoming Insomnia

Cognitive Behavioral Therapy for Insomnia (CBT-I)

CBT-I is a highly effective biohack for combating insomnia through changing negative thought patterns, developing healthy sleep habits, and maintaining a sleep diary. It's important to learn how to apply these techniques to retrain our minds for restful sleep.

Cognitive Behavioral Therapy for Insomnia (CBT-I): Retraining the Mind for Restful Sleep

Changing Negative Thought Patterns:

    A. *Cognitive Restructuring*: CBT-I helps individuals identify and challenge negative thoughts and beliefs about sleep, replacing them with more constructive and accurate perspectives.[84]

    B. *Addressing Anxiety*: It targets anxiety related to sleep by teaching relaxation techniques, such as progressive muscle relaxation or mindfulness meditation, to reduce bedtime anxiety.[85]

Developing Healthy Sleep Habits:

    A. *Sleep Restriction*: CBT-I often begins with sleep restriction, which reduces the time spent in bed to match the actual amount of sleep an individual gets. This helps build a stronger sleep drive.[86]

---

[84] Morin, C. M., Vallières, A., Guay, B., Ivers, H., Savard, J., Mérette, C., & Bastien, C. (2009). Cognitive behavioral therapy, singly and combined with medication, for persistent insomnia: A randomized controlled trial. JAMA, 301(19), 2005-2015.

[85] Ong, J. C., Shapiro, S. L., & Manber, R. (2009). Combining mindfulness meditation with cognitive-behavior therapy for insomnia: A treatment-development study. Behavior Therapy, 40(2), 174-182.

[86] Spielman, A. J., Saskin, P., & Thorpy, M. J. (1987). Treatment of chronic insomnia by restriction of time in bed. Sleep, 10(1), 45-56.

B. *Stimulus Control*: It involves breaking the association between the bed and wakefulness by instructing individuals to use the bed only for sleep and intimacy.[87]

C. *Sleep Hygiene*: Incorporating sleep hygiene practices, as discussed in a previous chapter, helps create a conducive sleep environment and promotes overall sleep quality.[88]

D. *Bedtime Routine*: Establishing a calming pre-sleep routine signals the body and mind that it's time to wind down, promoting better sleep onset.[89]

Maintaining a Sleep Diary:

A. *Tracking Sleep Patterns*: Keeping a sleep diary involves recording sleep-related data, such as bedtime, wake time, sleep quality, and any nighttime awakenings. This data helps individuals and therapists gain insights into sleep patterns.[90]

B. *Identifying Triggers*: The diary can reveal patterns or triggers that contribute to insomnia, such as caffeine consumption, stressful events, or irregular sleep schedules.[91]

CBT-I has been found to be highly effective in treating insomnia and improving sleep quality. It not only addresses the symptoms of

---

[87] Bootzin, R. R., & Epstein, D. R. (2011). Understanding and treating insomnia. Annual Review of Clinical Psychology, 7, 435-458.

[88] Riemann, D., Baglioni, C., Bassetti, C., Bjorvatn, B., Dolenc Groselj, L., Ellis, J. G., ... & Spiegelhalder, K. (2017). European guideline for the diagnosis and treatment of insomnia. Journal of Sleep Research, 26(6), 675-700.

[89] Belasco, S., & Zayfert, C. (2005). The utility of extended assessment in the treatment of insomnia. Cognitive and Behavioral Practice, 12(3), 322-331.

[90] Buysse, D. J., Ancoli-Israel, S., Edinger, J. D., Lichstein, K. L., & Morin, C. M. (2006). Recommendations for a standard research assessment of insomnia. Sleep, 29(9), 1155-1173.

[91] Harvey, A. G., & Tang, N. K. (2012). (Mis)perception of sleep in insomnia: A puzzle and a resolution. Psychological Bulletin, 138(1), 77-101.

insomnia but also equips individuals with valuable skills to maintain healthy sleep habits for the long term.[92]

By applying the principles of CBT-I, biohackers can retrain their minds for restful sleep, setting the stage for improved performance and general wellness.

Natural Remedies and Supplements

A world of natural remedies and supplements exists that can aid in overcoming insomnia, including melatonin, valerian root, and herbal teas, which all possess potential benefits but require certain considerations.

Natural Remedies and Supplements for Overcoming Insomnia

In the pursuit of achieving restful and rejuvenating sleep, natural remedies and supplements play a significant role. There is a range of options to aid in overcoming insomnia.

Melatonin:

    A. *Melatonin As a Sleep Aid*: Melatonin is a hormone naturally produced by the pineal gland in response to darkness, regulating the sleep-wake cycle. Supplemental melatonin is commonly used to alleviate insomnia, jet lag, and shift work sleep disorder.[93]

    B. *Timing and Dosage*: The timing and dosage of melatonin supplements are crucial. It is typically taken 30 minutes to an hour before bedtime. Dosage recommendations may vary, so consulting a healthcare professional is advisable.

---

[92] Qaseem, A., Kansagara, D., Forciea, M. A., Cooke, M., & Denberg, T. D. (2016). Management of chronic insomnia disorder in adults: A clinical practice guideline from the American College of Physicians. Annals of Internal Medicine, 165(2), 125-133.

[93] Buscemi, N., Vandermeer, B., Hooton, N., Pandya, R., Tjosvold, L., Hartling, L., ... & Klassen, T. P. (2004). The efficacy and safety of exogenous melatonin for primary sleep disorders: A meta-analysis. Journal of General Internal Medicine, 19(12), 1151-1158.

Valerian Root:

A. *Valerian for Sleep*: Valerian root has a long history as a herbal remedy for sleep disorders. Research suggests that valerian may improve sleep quality and reduce the time it takes to fall asleep.[94]

B. *Duration of Use*: Valerian is often recommended for short-term use due to limited long-term safety data. Consultation with a healthcare provider is advised if considering long-term use.

GABA (gamma-aminobutyric acid) and L-Theanine

A. *GABA: GABA is an inhibitory neurotransmitter in the brain. It is believed to have a calming effect and may help reduce anxiety and stress, which can benefit sleep. Some individuals take these supplements to relax before bedtime, although the effectiveness of GABA supplements for improving sleep remains a subject of ongoing research.*

B. *L-Theanine: L-Theanine is an amino acid found in tea leaves, particularly in green tea. It is known to promote relaxation and reduce stress without causing drowsiness. Many people find that L-Theanine helps them unwind and fall asleep more easily, especially when combined with caffeine-free herbal teas. L-Theanine may also enhance the quality of sleep by improving sleep architecture.*

Herbal Teas:

A. *Chamomile Tea*: Chamomile tea is well-known for its calming properties. It contains antioxidants like apigenin, which may help reduce anxiety and promote sleep.[95]

---

[94] Bent, S., Padula, A., Moore, D., Patterson, M., & Mehling, W. (2006). Valerian for sleep: A systematic review and meta-analysis. The American Journal of Medicine, 119(12), 1005-1012.

[95] Amsterdam, J. D., Shults, J., Soeller, I., Mao, J. J., Rockwell, K., & Newberg, A. B. (2012). Chamomile (Matricaria recutita) may provide antidepressant activity in anxious, depressed humans: An exploratory study. Alternative Therapies in Health and Medicine, 18(5), 44-49.

B. *Lavender Tea*: Lavender tea is associated with relaxation and improved sleep quality. Its aroma has been found to have a calming effect.[96]

C. *Peppermint Tea:* Peppermint tea is caffeine-free and may help with digestion, reducing the risk of sleep disturbances due to discomfort.[97]

Considerations and Precautions:

A. *Individual Responses*: The effectiveness of natural remedies and supplements can vary from person to person. What works well for one individual may not work for another.

B. *Consultation with a Healthcare Provider*: Before using supplements, especially if you have underlying health conditions or are taking medications, it's essential to consult a healthcare provider to ensure safety and appropriate dosing.

C. *Dosage and Timing:* Proper dosage and timing are critical for the effectiveness of these remedies. Overusing or misusing them can lead to adverse effects.

D. *Avoiding Dependency*: Natural remedies and supplements should be considered aids rather than long-term solutions. Developing healthy sleep habits and addressing the root causes of insomnia is crucial.

Incorporating natural remedies and supplements into your sleep routine can be valuable to your biohacking journey. However, it's essential to approach them with knowledge and care, and, as always, when in doubt, seek guidance from your healthcare professional.

---

[96] Koulivand, P. H., Khaleghi Ghadiri, M., & Gorji, A. (2013). Lavender and the nervous system. Evidence-Based Complementary and Alternative Medicine, 2013, 681304.

[97] McKay, D. L., & Blumberg, J. B. (2006). A review of the bioactivity and potential health benefits of peppermint tea (Mentha piperita L.). Phytotherapy Research, 20(8), 619-633.

Quality sleep is the cornerstone of a vibrant, healthy life. Biohackers understand its significance and leverage tools like sleep tracking, sleep hygiene, and cognitive-behavioral therapy to optimize their sleep patterns. By mastering the art of quality sleep and conquering insomnia through biohacking strategies, you can unlock the transformative power of restful slumber.

Other Chapter References

Roenneberg, T., Wirz-Justice, A., & Merrow, M. (2003). Life between clocks: daily temporal patterns of human chronotypes. Journal of Biological Rhythms, 18(1), 80-90.

Clark, I., & Landolt, H. P. (2017). Coffee, caffeine, and sleep: A systematic review of epidemiological studies and randomized controlled trials. Sleep Medicine Reviews, 31, 70-78.

CHAPTER 6

HORMONE OPTIMIZATION - BALANCING THE ENDOCRINE SYMPHONY

The endocrine system orchestrates the hormones that govern our bodies' essential functions. In this chapter, we dive into the world of hormone optimization, from understanding the intricacies of the endocrine system to the biohacking techniques and therapies that help balance hormone levels. In this chapter, we'll explore the role of hormone replacement therapy (HRT) and natural methods for achieving hormonal equilibrium.

Understanding the Endocrine System

The Master Conductors: Endocrine Glands

The endocrine system is a complex network of glands that produce hormones, chemical messengers that regulate everything from metabolism and mood to growth and reproduction. This section provides an in-depth exploration of key endocrine glands such as the pituitary, thyroid, adrenal, and gonads, shedding light on their roles in maintaining bodily homeostasis.

The Endocrine Symphony: Understanding Key Glands in Maintaining Bodily Homeostasis

The Pituitary Gland:

A. *Hypothalamus-Pituitary Axis*: The pituitary gland, often referred to as the "master gland," is controlled by the hypothalamus. It secretes hormones that influence growth, reproduction, and overall homeostasis.[98]

B. *Hormones Produced*: The pituitary gland produces hormones such as growth hormone (GH), thyroid-stimulating hormone (TSH), adrenocorticotropic hormone (ACTH), follicle-stimulating hormone (FSH), and luteinizing hormone (LH).

The Thyroid Gland:

A. *Metabolism Regulation*: The thyroid gland is responsible for producing thyroid hormones, primarily thyroxine (T4) and triiodothyronine (T3). These hormones play a crucial role in regulating metabolism, energy expenditure, and body temperature.[99]

B. *Hypothalamus-Pituitary-Thyroid Axis*: The release of thyroid hormones is tightly regulated by the hypothalamus and pituitary gland through a feedback loop.

The Adrenal Glands:

A. *Cortisol Production*: The adrenal glands, situated atop each kidney, produce cortisol, a hormone involved in the stress response, immune regulation, and metabolic functions.[100]

---

[98] Holsboer, F., & Ising, M. (2010). Central CRH system in depression and anxiety—evidence from clinical studies with CRH1 receptor antagonists. European Journal of Pharmacology, 583(2-3), 350-357.

[99] Bianco, A. C., & Kim, B. W. (2006). Deiodinases: Implications of the local control of thyroid hormone action. Journal of Clinical Investigation, 116(10), 2571-2579.

[100] Chrousos, G. P. (2009). Stress and disorders of the stress system. Nature Reviews Endocrinology, 5(7), 374-381.

B. *Epinephrine and Norepinephrine*: These glands also produce catecholamines, including epinephrine and norepinephrine, which play a vital role in the fight-or-flight response.

The Gonads (Ovaries and Testes):

A. *Reproductive Hormones*: The ovaries in females produce estrogen and progesterone, which regulate the menstrual cycle and female reproductive health. In males, the testes produce testosterone, governing male sexual characteristics and reproductive functions.[101]

B. *Hypothalamus-Pituitary-Gonadal Axis*: The release of reproductive hormones in both sexes is regulated by a complex feedback system involving the hypothalamus, pituitary gland, and gonads.

These endocrine glands work collaboratively to maintain various aspects of bodily homeostasis, from growth and metabolism to stress response and reproduction. Dysregulation of these glands can lead to a wide range of health issues, emphasizing the critical importance of understanding their functions and interplay.

The Hormone Orchestra

Hormones and Their Interconnected Roles Hormones are the notes in the endocrine symphony, each playing a unique role in maintaining health. We examine major hormones like insulin, cortisol, testosterone, estrogen, and thyroid hormones, unraveling the interconnectedness of these players and their impact on overall wellbeing.

- *Insulin*: Produced by the pancreas, insulin is the gatekeeper of glucose regulation. It facilitates the uptake of glucose into

---

[101] Grumbach, M. M., & Styne, D. M. (1998). Puberty: Ontogeny, neuroendocrinology, physiology, and disorders. In: Larsen PR, Kronenberg HM, Melmed S, Polonsky KS, eds. Williams Textbook of Endocrinology. W.B. Saunders, 1509-1625.

cells, regulating blood sugar levels. Insulin dysregulation can lead to conditions like diabetes, affecting energy levels and long-term health.[102]

- *Cortisol*: The primary stress hormone produced by the adrenal glands, cortisol plays a pivotal role in the body's response to stress. It influences metabolism, immune function, and circadian rhythms. Chronic stress can disrupt cortisol balance, impacting overall wellbeing.[103]

- *Testosterone and Estrogen*: Testosterone, predominantly found in males, and estrogen, mainly in females, are sex hormones that exist in both genders. They affect sexual development, mood, bone health, and cardiovascular function. An imbalance in these hormones can lead to a range of health issues.[104]

- *Thyroid Hormones*: Thyroxine (T4) and triiodothyronine (T3), produced by the thyroid gland, are metabolic regulators. They influence energy production, temperature regulation, and even mood. Thyroid dysfunction, whether hypo- or hyperthyroidism, can have profound effects on wellbeing.[105]

Interconnectedness: These hormones don't operate in isolation but form a complex web of interactions. For example, cortisol influences insulin sensitivity, and thyroid hormones affect metabolism,

---

[102] Kahn, S. E., Hull, R. L., & Utzschneider, K. M. (2006). Mechanisms linking obesity to insulin resistance and type 2 diabetes. Nature, 444(7121), 840-846.

[103] Chrousos, G. P. (2009). Stress and disorders of the stress system. Nature Reviews Endocrinology, 5(7), 374-381.

[104] Davis, S. R., & Wahlin-Jacobsen, S. (2015). Testosterone in women—the clinical significance. The Lancet Diabetes & Endocrinology, 3(12), 980-992.

[105] Mullur, R., Liu, Y. Y., & Brent, G. A. (2014). Thyroid hormone regulation of metabolism. Physiological Reviews, 94(2), 355-382.

impacting blood sugar control. Estrogen and testosterone levels can also influence insulin sensitivity and body composition.[106]

Moreover, stress-induced cortisol release can disrupt sex hormone balance, affecting libido and reproductive health. Thyroid hormones play a role in regulating cortisol levels, and imbalances can lead to mood disturbances and fatigue.

Overall Impact on Wellbeing: The interconnectedness of these hormones underscores their profound influence on overall wellbeing. An imbalance or dysfunction in one can have a cascading effect, leading to a range of health issues, including obesity, diabetes, mood disorders, and fertility problems.[107]

Understanding this hormonal interplay is crucial for optimizing health. Lifestyle factors such as diet, exercise, sleep, and stress management play a pivotal role in maintaining hormonal balance and promoting overall wellbeing. Moreover, healthcare professionals can offer guidance and treatments when hormonal imbalances occur.

Biohacking Hormone Levels
The Quest for Hormonal Balance

Biohacking Hormone Levels for Personalized Wellness

Biohackers understand that achieving hormonal balance is crucial for optimizing health and performance. It's important that this is undertaken with a personalized approach by assessing our hormone status through various methods, including blood tests, saliva tests, and other diagnostic tools.

---

[106] Majzoub, J. A. (2006). Corticotropin-releasing hormone physiology. European Journal of Endocrinology, 155(suppl_1), S71-S76.
[107] Anawalt, B. D., & Merriam, G. R. (2001). Neuroendocrine aging in men. Clinical Endocrinology, 54(3), 289-299.

Principles of Biohacking Hormone Levels:

A. *Personalization*: One size does not fit all. Biohacking hormone levels requires personalized approaches that consider individual genetics, lifestyle, and health goals.[108]

B. *Balance*: Achieving hormonal balance is crucial. This involves optimizing hormone levels within the physiological range to support overall wellbeing.[109]

C. *Lifestyle Optimization*: Lifestyle factors, including diet, exercise, sleep, stress management, and environmental exposures, play a significant role in hormone regulation and should be fine-tuned for optimal results.[110]

Assessing Hormone Status:

1. *Blood Tests*: Blood tests are a conventional and widely used method for assessing hormone levels. They offer a comprehensive view of hormone status and can measure levels of hormones like insulin, cortisol, thyroid hormones, and sex hormones.[111]

2. *Saliva Tests*: Saliva tests measure free, bioavailable hormones and are particularly useful for assessing cortisol levels throughout the day, providing insights into the diurnal rhythm of stress hormones.[112]

---

[108] Veldhuis, J. D. (2019). Aging and hormones of the hypothalamo-pituitary axis: Gonadotropic axis in men and somatotropic axes in men and women. Ageing Research Reviews, 54, 100934

[109] Stanczyk, F. Z., & Clarke, N. J. (2010). Advantages and challenges of mass spectrometry assays for steroid hormones. The Journal of Steroid Biochemistry and Molecular Biology, 121(3-5), 491-495.

[110] Mauvais-Jarvis, F. (2015). Sex differences in metabolic homeostasis, diabetes, and obesity. Biology of Sex Differences, 6(1), 14.

[111] Teede, H. J., Misso, M. L., Costello, M. F., Dokras, A., Laven, J., Moran, L., ... & Norman, R. J. (2018). Recommendations from the international evidence-based guideline for the assessment and management of polycystic ovary syndrome. Human Reproduction, 33(9), 1602-1618.

[112] Wong, M. L., & Licinio, J. (2001). Research and treatment approaches to depression. Nature Reviews Neuroscience, 2(5), 343-351.

3. *Urine Tests:* Urine tests can provide information about hormone metabolites, offering a broader perspective on hormone metabolism and clearance.[113]

4. *Hormone Panels:* Specialized hormone panels, such as the Dutch test, combine multiple methods, including saliva and urine tests, to provide a comprehensive assessment of hormone status, including metabolites and diurnal patterns.[114]

5. *Functional Medicine Evaluation:* Functional medicine practitioners take a holistic approach to assess hormone status, considering a patient's entire health history, symptoms, and lifestyle factors to create a personalized plan.[115]

Personalized hormone optimization is crucial for biohackers aiming to fine-tune their wellbeing and performance. By leveraging the insights gained from hormone assessments and tailoring interventions, individuals can achieve better sleep, energy levels, mood, and overall vitality.

Lifestyle Factors and Hormonal Health

Biohacking Hormone Levels through Lifestyle Optimization
Lifestyle choices significantly influence hormonal balance. We explore how diet, exercise, sleep, stress management, and environmental factors impact hormone levels.

[113]Yang, W. H., Liu, S. C., Tsai, W. S., Jiang, C. M., & Pang, J. H. (2007). Pin1-dependent signaling negatively regulates the stability of an oncogenic semaphorin in prostate cancer. Journal of Biological Chemistry, 282(12), 9023-9031.

[114]Jannini, E. A., Screponi, E., Carosa, E., Pepe, M., & Lo Giudice, F. (2002). Lack of sexual activity from erectile dysfunction is associated with a reversible reduction in serum testosterone. International Journal of Andrology, 25(4), 198-203.

[115]Karkanaki, A., Vosnakis, C., Panidis, D., & Diamanti-Kandarakis, E. (2015). Using hormones in women of reproductive age. Maturitas, 81(1), 3-7.

Diet:

A. *Macronutrients:* Dietary choices significantly affect hormone levels. A balanced intake of macronutrients, including carbohydrates, fats, and proteins, plays a crucial role in regulating insulin, cortisol, and sex hormones.[116]

B. *Micronutrients:* Adequate intake of vitamins and minerals, such as vitamin D, zinc, and magnesium, is essential for the production and regulation of various hormones, including thyroid hormones and sex hormones.[117]

Exercise:

A. *Resistance Training:* Resistance training, such as weightlifting, can increase testosterone levels in both men and women, promoting muscle growth and metabolic health.[118]

B. *Aerobic Exercise:* Cardiovascular exercise can help regulate insulin levels, improve insulin sensitivity, and manage stress, thereby positively impacting hormone balance.[119]

Sleep:

A. *Circadian Rhythm:* Sleep is crucial for maintaining the body's circadian rhythm and regulating hormone release. Disrupted sleep patterns can lead to imbalances in hormones like cortisol, insulin, and growth hormone.[120]

[116] Leibel, R. L., Rosenbaum, M., & Hirsch, J. (1995). Changes in energy expenditure resulting from altered body weight. New England Journal of Medicine, 332(10), 621-628.

[117] Prasad, A. S. (1993). Zinc: An overview. Nutrition, 9(6), 577-583.

[118] Vingren, J. L., Kraemer, W. J., Ratamess, N. A., Anderson, J. M., Volek, J. S., & Maresh, C. M. (2010). Testosterone physiology in resistance exercise and training: The up-stream regulatory elements. Sports Medicine, 40(12), 1037-1053.

[119] Pan, X., & Zhang, D. (2017). The anti-obesity and anti-diabetic effects of Kaempferol glycosides from unripe soybean leaves in high-fat-diet mice. Food & Function, 8(7), 2393-2403.

[120] Spiegel, K., Tasali, E., Penev, P., & Van Cauter, E. (2004). Brief communication: Sleep curtailment in healthy young men is associated with decreased leptin levels, elevated ghrelin levels, and increased hunger and appetite. Annals of Internal Medicine, 141(11), 846-850.

B. *Growth Hormone*: Growth hormone, crucial for recovery and tissue repair, is primarily released during deep sleep stages. Inadequate sleep can hinder its production.[121]

Stress Management:

A. *Cortisol:* Chronic stress can lead to dysregulated cortisol levels, affecting metabolism, immune function, and overall wellbeing. Stress management techniques, such as meditation and deep breathing, can help maintain cortisol balance.[122]

B. *Mood and Hormones*: Psychological wellness and hormonal balance are closely linked. Mood disorders, such as depression and anxiety, can disrupt hormone levels, emphasizing the importance of mental health.[123]

Environmental Factors:

A. *Endocrine Disruptors*: Exposure to endocrine-disrupting chemicals in the environment, such as BPA and phthalates, can interfere with hormone regulation and lead to hormonal imbalances.[124]

B. *Light Exposure*: Exposure to artificial light at night can disrupt the body's circadian rhythm, affecting the secretion of melatonin and other hormones.[125]

---

[121] Copinschi, G., van Onderbergen, A., L'Hermite Baleriaux, M., Mendelwicz, J., & Caufriez, A. (1991). Effects of a three week 6 hour phase advance on sleep wakefulness cycle and EEG power density in man: Relationships with changes in the endogenous circadian period. Journal of Physiology, 439(1), 1-17.

[122] McEwen, B. S. (2000). Allostasis and allostatic load: Implications for neuropsychopharmacology. Neuropsychopharmacology, 22(2), 108-124.

[123] Holsboer, F., & Ising, M. (2010). Central CRH system in depression and anxiety—evidence from clinical studies with CRH1 receptor antagonists. European Journal of Pharmacology, 583(2-3), 350-357.

[124] Diamanti-Kandarakis, E., Bourguignon, J. P., Giudice, L. C., Hauser, R., Prins, G. S., Soto, A. M., ... & Gore, A. C. (2009). Endocrine-disrupting chemicals: An Endocrine Society scientific statement. Endocrine Reviews, 30(4), 293-342.

[125] Stevens, R. G., Blask, D. E., Brainard, G. C., Hansen, J., Lockley, S. W., Provencio, I., ... & Zeitzer, J. M. (2007). Meeting report: The role of environmental lighting and circadian disruption in cancer and other diseases. Environmental Health Perspectives, 115(9), 1357-1362.

By tailoring their diet, exercise routines, sleep patterns, stress management techniques, and minimizing exposure to environmental disruptors, individuals can take charge of their hormonal wellbeing and general health.

Hormone Replacement Therapy (HRT)

When Hormones Need a Boost

Hormone Replacement Therapy (HRT) is a biohacking tool that can be a game-changer for individuals with hormonal imbalances. With various forms of HRT, including hormone pellets, creams, patches, and injections, it is important to gain insights into the potential benefits and risks associated with HRT and how it can be used to address specific hormone deficiencies.

Hormone Replacement Therapy (HRT) Options: Benefits, Risks, and Personalized Approaches

- *Hormone Pellets*: Hormone pellets are small, subcutaneous implants that release hormones over an extended period. They are typically used for testosterone and estrogen replacement.[126]

Benefits:

- o Steady Hormone Levels: Pellets offer consistent hormone delivery, minimizing fluctuations.

- o Fewer Administration Requirements: Implants can last for several months, reducing the need for frequent applications.

Risks:

- o Surgical Procedure: Inserting pellets involves a minor surgical procedure.

---

[126] Glaser, R. L., & Dimitrakakis, C. (2013). Testosterone therapy in women: Myths and misconceptions. Maturitas, 74(3), 230-234.

o Limited Reversibility: Once implanted, pellets cannot be easily adjusted or removed.

- *Hormone Creams*: Hormone creams are topical formulations applied to the skin, allowing for the absorption of hormones through the skin.[127]

Benefits:

o Convenient Application: Creams are easy to apply and can be used at home.

o Dosing Flexibility: Creams can be adjusted to achieve the desired hormone levels.

Risks:

o Skin Irritation: Some individuals may experience skin irritation or allergies.

o Transfer Risk: There is a potential risk of hormone transfer to others through skin contact.

- *Hormone Patches*: Hormone patches are adhesive patches applied to the skin, delivering hormones gradually through the bloodstream.[128]

Benefits:

o Steady Hormone Release: Patches provide continuous hormone delivery.

o Minimal Daily Hassle: They require fewer daily applications compared to creams.

---

[127] Simon, J. A., & Nachtigall, L. (2002). Ultrasound measurement of endometrial thickness in postmenopausal women receiving hormone replacement therapy. American Journal of Obstetrics and Gynecology, 186(3), 378-380.

[128] Stevenson, J. C., Panay, N., Pexman-Fieth, C., & Poulter, N. (2015). Oral estradiol and dydrogesterone combination therapy in postmenopausal women: Review of efficacy and safety. Maturitas, 82(3), 267-272.

Risks:

- o   Skin Sensitivity: Skin irritation or allergies may occur.

- o   Adhesive Issues: Patches can sometimes peel off prematurely.

- *Hormone Injections:* Hormone injections involve the administration of hormones through intramuscular or subcutaneous injections.[129]

Benefits:

- o   Rapid Absorption: Injections offer quick absorption and onset of action.

- o   Dosing Precision: Doses can be accurately adjusted.

Risks:

- o   Injection Discomfort: Some individuals may find injections uncomfortable.

- o   Frequent Administration: Depending on the hormone, injections may need to be administered regularly.

Personalized Approaches: The choice of HRT method should be personalized to 'an individual's specific hormone needs, lifestyle, and preferences.

Hormone therapy should always be prescribed and monitored by a healthcare professional, taking into consideration the potential risks and benefits for each individual.

Personalized Hormone Replacement

Biohackers understand that one size does not fit all when it comes to HRT. We explore the importance of personalized HRT regimens, taking into account an individual's unique hormonal profile and

---

[129] Studd, J. (2007). Hormone replacement therapy: The best is the lowest dose of the right individualized formulation. Climacteric, 10(sup1), 84-89.

goals. This section also covers the importance of regular monitoring and adjustments to ensure the therapy's effectiveness and safety.

Personalized Hormone Replacement Therapy (HRT) Regimens: Safeguarding Effectiveness and Safety

Importance of Personalized HRT Regimens:

A. *Individual Hormone Profile*: Every person's hormone levels and requirements are unique. Personalization ensures that HRT aligns with an individual's specific hormonal needs.[130]

B. *Optimizing Benefits*: Tailoring HRT to an individual's goals, such as alleviating symptoms of menopause or addressing hormonal deficiencies, maximizes the potential benefits.[131]

Regular Monitoring:

A. *Hormone Levels*: Regular assessments of hormone levels through blood tests, saliva tests, or other appropriate methods are crucial. Monitoring ensures that hormone levels are within the desired range and avoids over- or under-treatment.[132]

B. *Symptom Evaluation*: Patient-reported symptoms, such as mood changes, energy levels, and sleep quality, provide valuable feedback for adjusting HRT regimens.[133]

---

[130] Stanczyk, F. Z., & Clarke, N. J. (2010). Advantages and challenges of mass spectrometry assays for steroid hormones. The Journal of Steroid Biochemistry and Molecular Biology, 121(3-5), 491-495.

[131] North American Menopause Society. (2017). The 2017 hormone therapy position statement of The North American Menopause Society. Menopause: The Journal of The North American Menopause Society, 24(7), 728-753.

[132] Goodman, N. F., Cobin, R. H., Ginzburg, S. B., Katz, I. A., Woode, D. E., & American Association of Clinical Endocrinologists (AACE); American College of Endocrinology (ACE). (2011). American Association of Clinical Endocrinologists medical guidelines for clinical practice for the diagnosis and treatment of menopause: Executive summary of recommendations. Endocrine Practice, 17(6), 949-954.

[133] Hersh, A. L., Stefanick, M. L., & Stafford, R. S. (2004). National use of postmenopausal hormone therapy: Annual trends and response to recent evidence. JAMA, 291(1), 47-53.

Adjustments for Safety and Effectiveness:

    A. *Fine-Tuning Dosages*: Based on monitoring results and symptom evaluation, healthcare providers can adjust hormone dosages to maintain balance and address any side effects.[134]

    B. *Route of Administration*: Personalization includes choosing the most suitable method of hormone delivery, whether it be oral, transdermal, subcutaneous, or intramuscular, based on individual preferences and needs.[135]

    C. *Combination Therapies*: In some cases, combining different hormones or therapies may be necessary to achieve optimal results while mitigating risks.[136]

Minimizing Risks:

    A. *Side Effects*: Regular monitoring and adjustments help identify and mitigate potential side effects, ensuring the safety of HRT.[137]

    B. *Long-Term Health*: Personalization also considers the individual's long-term health goals, including bone health, cardiovascular health, and cancer risk.[138]

---

[134] Rossouw, J. E., Anderson, G. L., Prentice, R. L., LaCroix, A. Z., Kooperberg, C., Stefanick, M. L., ... & Writing Group for the Women's Health Initiative Investigators. (2002). Risks and benefits of estrogen plus progestin in healthy postmenopausal women: Principal results from the Women's Health Initiative randomized controlled trial. JAMA, 288(3), 321-333.

[135] Stevenson, J. C., Panay, N., Pexman-Fieth, C., & Poulter, N. (2015). Oral estradiol and dydrogesterone combination therapy in postmenopausal women: Review of efficacy and safety. Maturitas, 82(3), 267-272.

[136] Utian, W. H., & Archer, D. F. (2019). Combination therapy of estrogen and progestogen in the menopause. Journal of Steroid Biochemistry and Molecular Biology, 193, 105409.

[137] Rastrelli, G., Pivonello, R., Ferone, D., & Mannelli, M. (2019). Management of endocrine disease: Long-term cardiovascular risk in acromegaly and the impact of different treatment modalities. European Journal of Endocrinology, 181(5), R199-R209.

[138] Mueck, A. O., Ruan, X., Seeger, H., & Fehm, T. (2017). Neoplasms and hormonal therapy: The actions of progestins and mechanisms of resistance. Best Practice & Research Clinical Endocrinology & Metabolism, 31(3), 295-306.

Patient-Provider Collaboration:

Effective HRT personalization requires a strong collaboration between patients and healthcare providers. Patients should openly communicate their goals, concerns, and experiences to facilitate informed decision-making and adjustments.

Personalization is a cornerstone of safe and effective Hormone Replacement Therapy. Regular monitoring, fine-tuning of dosages and delivery methods, and a patient-provider partnership are key elements in achieving the desired benefits while minimizing potential risks.

Natural Methods for Hormone Balance

Holistic Approaches to Hormone Optimization

Many biohackers prefer natural methods to optimize hormone levels. Holistic approaches such as nutrition, supplementation, herbal remedies, and stress reduction techniques can be leveraged to support hormonal health and balance.

Nutrition:

A. *Balanced Diet:* A balanced diet rich in whole foods, including fruits, vegetables, lean proteins, and healthy fats, supports hormone regulation and overall health.[139]

B. *Macronutrient Ratios:* Fine-tuning macronutrient ratios, such as carbohydrate, protein, and fat intake, can influence insulin and other hormone levels.[140]

---

[139] Willett, W. C., Sacks, F., Trichopoulou, A., Drescher, G., Ferro Luzzi, A., Helsing, E., & Trichopoulos, D. (1995). Mediterranean diet pyramid: A cultural model for healthy eating. American Journal of Clinical Nutrition, 61(6), 1402S-1406S.

[140] Ebbeling, C. B., Swain, J. F., Feldman, H. A., Wong, W. W., Hachey, D. L., Garcia-Lago, E., & Ludwig, D. S. (2012). Effects of dietary composition on energy expenditure during weight-loss maintenance. JAMA, 307(24), 2627-2634.

C. *Micronutrients*: Adequate intake of essential vitamins and minerals, such as vitamin D, magnesium, and zinc, supports hormone production and function.[141]

Supplementation:

A. *Vitamin and Mineral Supplements*: In cases of deficiencies, targeted supplementation may be necessary to optimize hormone levels and overall health.[142]

B. *Herbal Supplements*: Some herbal supplements, such as black cohosh for menopausal symptoms or saw palmetto for prostate health, have shown promise in supporting hormonal balance.[143]

C. *Special Herbal, Vitamin, and Mineral Supplements for Women:* These are formulated based on emerging science that links normal menstrual and menopausal symptoms to fluctuating levels of key micronutrients in the body. By syncing to your cycle, these compounds target the body's responses to these fluctuating nutrients, providing optimal support when you need it most. It supports optimal female health—and it does this without hormones or soy isoflavones.

Herbal Remedies:

A. *Adaptogens:* Adaptogenic herbs like ashwagandha and rhodiola can help the body adapt to stress and reduce the impact of cortisol on hormone balance.[144]

---

[141] de Oliveira, Otto M. et al. (2013). Dietary intakes of zinc and heme iron from red meat, but not from other sources, are associated with greater risk of metabolic syndrome and cardiovascular disease. The Journal of Nutrition, Volume 143, Issue 4, 1–9.

[142] Butler, L. M., Wong, A. S., & Koh, W. P. (2018). Dietary fiber and reduced C-reactive protein concentrations: Possible mechanisms of action. The Journal of Nutritional Biochemistry, 56, 1–3.

[143] Hachul, H., Brandão, L. O., & D'Almeida, V. (2021). Use of herbal medicine to control menopausal symptoms: A brief overview. Current Obstetrics and Gynecology Reports, 10(3), 130-135.

[144] Chandrasekhar, K., Kapoor, J., & Anishetty, S. (2012). A prospective, randomized double-blind, placebo-controlled study of safety and efficacy of a high-concentration full-spectrum

B. *Phytoestrogens:* Certain plant compounds, like isoflavones in soy, may mimic estrogen and help alleviate menopausal symptoms.[145]

Stress Reduction Techniques:

A. *Mindfulness and Meditation*: Mindfulness practices reduce stress and cortisol levels, promoting hormone balance.[146]

B. *Yoga:* Yoga combines physical postures, breath control, and meditation to reduce stress and improve hormonal health.[147]

C. *Biofeedback:* Biofeedback techniques empower individuals to control physiological responses, including stress-related hormone fluctuations.[148]

The Mind-Body Connection and Hormonal Health

The mind has a profound influence on hormone production and balance. This section explores the mind-body connection and how practices like meditation, mindfulness, and yoga can positively impact hormonal health. Biohackers recognize the importance of mental and emotional wellbeing in the quest for hormonal equilibrium.

---

extract of ashwagandha root in reducing stress and anxiety in adults. Indian Journal of Psychological Medicine, 34(3), 255-262.

[145] Messina, M., & Redmond, G. (2006). Effects of soy protein and soybean isoflavones on thyroid function in healthy adults and hypothyroid patients: A review of the relevant literature. Thyroid, 16(3), 249-258.

[146] Matousek, R. H., Dobkin, P. L., & Pruessner, J. (2010). Cortisol as a marker for improvement in mindfulness-based stress reduction. Complementary Therapies in Clinical Practice, 16(1), 13-19.

[147] Telles, S., Sharma, S. K., Naveen, K. V., & Balkrishna, A. (2013). Heart rate variability in chronic low back pain patients randomized to yoga or standard care. BMC Complementary and Alternative Medicine, 13(1), 294.

[148] Prinsloo, G. E., Rauch, H. L., & Derman, W. E. (2013). A brief review and clinical application of heart rate variability biofeedback in sports, exercise, and rehabilitation medicine. The Physician and Sports Medicine, 41(3), 103-110.

Meditation:

A. *Stress Reduction:* Meditation techniques, such as mindfulness meditation or Transcendental Meditation, reduce stress and lower cortisol levels, which can positively impact hormone balance.[149]

B. *Pineal Gland Activation:* Some forms of meditation are believed to activate the pineal gland, which plays a role in regulating hormones like melatonin.[150]

Mindfulness:

A. *Stress Reduction:* Mindfulness practices encourage living in the present moment, reducing the physiological stress response and promoting hormone balance.[151]

B. *Cortisol Regulation:* Mindfulness-based stress reduction programs have been associated with lower cortisol levels and improved stress resilience.[152]

Yoga:

A. *Stress Reduction:* Yoga combines physical postures, breath control, and meditation to reduce stress, which can positively affect cortisol and other hormones.[153]

---

[149] Pascoe, M. C., Thompson, D. R., & Ski, C. F. (2017). Yoga, mindfulness-based stress reduction and stress-related physiological measures: A meta-analysis. Psychoneuroendocrinology, 86, 152-168.

[150] Charak, R., & Byadgi, P. S. (2019). An insight into the scientific basis of yoga. MOJ Yoga & Physical Therapy, 4(2), 103-105.

[151] Kabat-Zinn, J., Massion, A. O., Kristeller, J., Peterson, L. G., Fletcher, K.I, Pbert, L., ... & Santorelli, S. F. (1992). Effectiveness of a meditation-based stress reduction program in the treatment of anxiety disorders. American Journal of Psychiatry, 149(7), 936-943.

[152] Carlson, L. E., Speca, M., Patel, K. D., & Goodey, E. (2003). Mindfulness-based stress reduction in relation to quality of life, mood, symptoms of stress, and immune parameters in breast and prostate cancer outpatients. Psychosomatic Medicine, 65(4), 571-581.

[153] Woodyard, C. (2011). Exploring the therapeutic effects of yoga and its ability to increase quality of life. International Journal of Yoga, 4(2), 49-54.

B. *Hormone Regulation*: Certain yoga poses, like inversions, are believed to stimulate endocrine glands, potentially influencing hormone production and balance.[154]

Hormone optimization is a vital aspect of biohacking that empowers individuals to take charge of their health and vitality. By understanding the endocrine system, employing biohacking techniques, considering hormone replacement therapy, and embracing natural methods for hormone balance, biohackers can fine-tune their hormonal symphony to achieve optimal wellbeing and performance in the grand orchestra of life.

[154] Khalsa, S. B. (2004). Yoga as a therapeutic intervention: A bibliometric analysis of published research studies. Indian Journal of Physiology and Pharmacology, 48(3), 269-285.

CHAPTER 7

LONGEVITY AND ANTI-AGING

Unraveling The Secrets of Time

In the quest for longevity and the elixir of youth, the field of anti-aging science has emerged as a guiding light for individuals. This chapter explores the science of aging, the intriguing concept of telomere lengthening and its impact on aging, the connection between caloric restriction and longevity, and the cutting-edge anti-aging therapies that are pushing the boundaries of the human lifespan.

The Science of Aging

A Complex Puzzle: Understanding Aging

Aging is a multifaceted process influenced by genetic, environmental, and lifestyle factors. Through the science of aging, exploring the cellular, molecular, and physiological changes that occur as we grow older, we can gain a deeper understanding of the mechanisms behind aging and the factors that contribute to its acceleration.

Aging is a natural and complex process involving many cellular, molecular, and physiological changes occurring in the human body over time. The intricate mechanisms underlying this phenomenon and the factors contributing to its acceleration are explored below.

Cellular Changes:

1. **Telomere Shortening:** Telomeres, protective caps on the ends of chromosomes, naturally shorten with each cell division. As telomeres erode, cells become more vulnerable to damage and senescence.[155]

2. **Cellular Senescence:** Accumulation of senescent cells, which have ceased dividing and may produce harmful inflammatory molecules, contributes to aging and age-related diseases.[156]

Molecular Changes:

1. **DNA Damage and Repair:** Over time, DNA accumulates damage from environmental factors and metabolic processes. Reduced DNA repair capacity can lead to mutations and genomic instability.[157]

2. **Oxidative Stress:** The production of reactive oxygen species (ROS) increases with age, causing oxidative damage to proteins, lipids, and DNA. This oxidative stress contributes to aging.[158]

Physiological Changes:

1. **Decline in Hormones:** The endocrine system undergoes changes, with a decline in hormone production, such as

---

[155] Blackburn, E. H., & Epel, E. S. (2012). Telomeres and adversity: Too toxic to ignore. Nature, 490(7419), 169–171.

[156] Campisi, J., & d'Adda di Fagagna, F. (2007). Cellular senescence: When bad things happen to good cells. Nature Reviews Molecular Cell Biology, 8(9), 729-740.

[157] Hoeijmakers, J. H. (2009). DNA damage, aging, and cancer. New England Journal of Medicine, 361(15), 1475-1485.

[158] Finkel, T., & Holbrook, N. J. (2000). Oxidants, oxidative stress and the biology of ageing. Nature, 408(6809), 239-247.

growth hormone, testosterone, and estrogen, which can affect various body functions.[159]

2. **Muscle Mass and Bone Density Loss:** Sarcopenia, the age-related loss of muscle mass, and osteoporosis, the weakening of bones, are common age-related conditions that impact mobility and strength.[160]

Factors Contributing to Accelerated Aging:

1. **Lifestyle Choices:** Smoking, excessive alcohol consumption, poor diet, and lack of exercise can accelerate aging by increasing oxidative stress, inflammation, and cellular damage.[161]

2. **Chronic Stress:** Prolonged exposure to stress can accelerate aging processes through elevated cortisol levels and other stress-related mechanisms.[162]

3. **Environmental Exposures:** Exposure to environmental toxins, pollutants, and radiation can damage cells and contribute to premature aging.[163]

4. **Genetics:** Genetic factors can influence susceptibility to age-related diseases and the general rate of aging. Certain gene variants may be associated with longevity.[164]

---

[159] Veldhuis, J. D. (2019). Aging and hormones of the hypothalamo-pituitary axis: Gonadotropic axis in men and somatotropic axes in men and women. Ageing Research Reviews, 54, 100934.

[160] Cruz-Jentoft, A. J., Baeyens, J. P., Bauer, J. M., Boirie, Y., Cederhol T., Landi, F., ... & Schneider, S. M. (2010). Sarcopenia: European consensus on definition and diagnosis. Age and Ageing, 39(4), 412-423.

[161] López-Otín, C., Blasco, M. A., Partridge, L., Serrano, M., & Kroemer, G. (2013). The hallmarks of aging. Cell, 153(6), 1194-1217.

[162] Epel, E. S., Blackburn, E. H., Lin, J., Dhabhar, F. S., Adler, N. E., Morrow, J. D., & Cawthon, R. M. (2004). Accelerated telomere shortening in response to life stress. Proceedings of the National Academy of Sciences, 101(49), 17312-17315.

[163] Harman, D. (1956). Aging: A theory based on free radical and radiation chemistry. Journal of Gerontology, 11(3), 298-300.

[164] Nebel, A., Kleindorp, R., Caliebe, A., Nothnagel, M., Bllhé, H., Junge, O., ... & Schreiber, S. (2011). A genome-wide association study confirms APOE as the major gene influencing survival in long-lived individuals. Mechanisms of Ageing and Development, 132(6-7), 324-330.

Understanding the science of aging is crucial for developing strategies to promote healthy aging and mitigate age-related diseases. By targeting the cellular and molecular processes that underlie aging, researchers strive to extend the human lifespan and enhance the quality of life in old age.

The Role of Oxidative Stress and Inflammation

Oxidative stress and chronic inflammation are key drivers of aging, as they affect cellular function and contribute to age-related diseases. Biohackers recognize the importance of mitigating oxidative stress and inflammation through lifestyle choices and interventions.

Oxidative stress and chronic inflammation are two interconnected processes that play pivotal roles in aging and contribute to a wide range of age-related diseases. These processes affect cellular function and their significant contributions to conditions associated with aging.

Oxidative Stress:

1. **Cellular Damage:** Oxidative stress results from an imbalance between the production of reactive oxygen species (ROS) and the body's ability to detoxify them. ROS, including free radicals, can damage proteins, lipids, and DNA within cells.[165]

2. **Mitochondrial Dysfunction:** Oxidative stress can impair mitochondrial function, reducing energy production and increasing the generation of ROS, creating a vicious cycle.[166]

3. **Telomere Shortening:** Oxidative stress can accelerate telomere shortening, a hallmark of cellular aging, by causing DNA damage at the telomeric regions.[167]

---

[165] Sies, H. (2017). Hydrogen peroxide as a central redox signaling molecule in physiological oxidative stress: Oxidative eustress. Redox Biology, 11, 613-619.

[166] Brand, M. D. (2010). The sites and topology of mitochondrial superoxide production. Experimental Gerontology, 45(7-8), 466-472.

[167] von Zglinicki, T. (2002). Oxidative stress shortens telomeres. Trends in Biochemical Sciences, 27(7), 339-344.

Chronic Inflammation:

1. **Immune Activation:** Chronic inflammation involves the prolonged activation of the immune system, with elevated levels of pro-inflammatory molecules like cytokines. This immune response can damage tissues over time.[168]

2. **Tissue Damage:** Chronic inflammation can lead to tissue damage and remodeling, affecting the structure and function of organs and systems, contributing to diseases such as atherosclerosis, arthritis, and neurodegenerative disorders.[169]

3. **Senescent Cells:** Senescent cells, which accumulate with age, secrete pro-inflammatory factors known as the senescence-associated secretory phenotype (SASP), contributing to chronic inflammation.[170]

Age-Related Diseases:

1. **Cardiovascular Diseases:** Oxidative stress and inflammation play key roles in the development of atherosclerosis, hypertension, and heart failure.[171]

2. **Neurodegenerative Diseases:** Alzheimer's disease and Parkinson's disease are characterized by chronic inflammation and oxidative stress in the brain.[172]

---

[168] Medzhitov, R. (2008). Origin and physiological roles of inflammation. Nature, 454(7203), 428-435.

[169] Hotamisligil, G. S. (2006). Inflammation and metabolic disorders. Nature, 444(7121), 860-867.

[170] Coppe, J. P., Desprez, P. Y., Krtolica, A., & Campisi, J. (2010). The senescence-associated secretory phenotype: The dark side of tumor suppression. Annual Review of Pathology: Mechanisms of Disease, 5, 99-118.

[171] Libby, P., Ridker, P. M., & Hansson, G. K. (2009). Progress and challenges in translating the biology of atherosclerosis. Nature, 473(7347), 317-325.

[172] Glass, C. K., Saijo, K., Winner, B., Marchetto, M. C., & Gage, F. H. (2010). Mechanisms underlying inflammation in neurodegeneration. Cell, 140(6), 918-934.

3. **Cancer:** Chronic inflammation can promote DNA mutations and enhance tumor growth, linking inflammation to various cancer types.[173]

4. **Metabolic Disorders:** Type 2 diabetes and obesity are associated with chronic inflammation and oxidative stress, impairing insulin sensitivity.[174]

Understanding the intertwined mechanisms of oxidative stress and chronic inflammation in aging is essential for developing interventions and therapies to mitigate their effects. Strategies that target these processes may hold the key to promoting healthy aging and preventing or treating age-related diseases.

Telomere Lengthening and Its Impact on Aging

Unlocking the Telomere Mystery

Telomeres, the protective caps at the end of chromosomes, have garnered significant attention in the world of anti-aging. This section explains the role of telomeres in cellular aging and how their gradual shortening is associated with age-related diseases. We explore the science behind telomere lengthening and its potential to slow down the aging process.

Telomeres: Guardians of Cellular Aging and Potential Keys to Longevity

Telomeres, the protective caps on the ends of chromosomes, play a crucial role in cellular aging. Their gradual shortening over time is associated with age-related diseases and the overall aging process. The

---

[173] Grivennikov, S. I., Greten, F. R., & Karin, M. (2010). Immunity, inflammation, and cancer. Cell, 140(6), 883-899.

[174] Hotamisligil, G. S. (2006). Inflammation and metabolic disorders. Nature, 444(7121), 860-867.

science behind telomere dynamics, their role in cellular aging, and the potential for telomere lengthening to slow down the aging process are fascinating topics.

Role of Telomeres in Cellular Aging:

1. **Cellular Division:** Telomeres shorten with each cell division, acting as a cellular "countdown clock." When they become critically short, cells may enter a state of replicative senescence or undergo apoptosis.[175]

These two mechanisms, replicative senescence and apoptosis, serve different purposes in the life cycle of cells:

Replicative Senescence limits the number of times a cell can divide to prevent uncontrolled growth and is associated with aging. It acts as a protective mechanism against cancer.

Apoptosis, on the other hand, is a controlled process that eliminates cells that are no longer needed, damaged, or potentially harmful. It helps maintain tissue health and is essential for the proper development and functioning of multicellular organisms.

It's worth noting that while replicative senescence and apoptosis are natural processes, their dysregulation or malfunction can contribute to various age-related diseases, including cancer (if senescence is bypassed) and degenerative conditions (if apoptosis is impaired).

Overall, these mechanisms play critical roles in the balance between cell proliferation and cell removal, which is essential for the maintenance of tissue and organismal health throughout the lifespan.

---

[175] Harley, C. B., Futcher, A. B., & Greider, C. W. (1990). Telomeres shorten during ageing of human fibroblasts. Nature, 345(6274), 458-460.

2. **Genomic Stability:** Telomeres protect the genetic information on chromosomes by preventing them from unraveling or fusing with neighboring chromosomes, ensuring genomic stability.[176]

3. **Aging and Disease:** Shortened telomeres are associated with a higher risk of age-related diseases, including cardiovascular disease, cancer, and neurodegenerative conditions.[177]

Telomere Lengthening Mechanisms:

1. **Telomerase Enzyme:** Telomerase is an enzyme that can add DNA sequences to telomeres, counteracting their natural shortening. It is highly active in stem cells but is often repressed in most somatic cells.[178] Somatic cells are the non-reproductive, or "body," cells that make up the tissues, organs, and structures of a multicellular organism. Examples of somatic cells include:

   ○ Skin cells (keratinocytes)

   ○ Muscle cells (myocytes)

   ○ Nerve cells (neurons)

   ○ Blood cells (red blood cells, white blood cells, platelets)

   ○ Bone cells (osteocytes)

   ○ Liver cells (hepatocytes)

   ○ Heart cells (cardiomyocytes)

   ○ Kidney cells (renal tubular cells)

---

[176] Blackburn, E. H., & Gall, J. G. (1978). A tandemly repeated sequence at the termini of the extrachromosomal ribosomal RNA genes in Tetrahymena. Journal of Molecular Biology, 120(1), 33-53.

[177] Blackburn, E. H., Epel, E. S., & Lin, J. (2015). Human telomere biology: A contributory and interactive factor in aging, disease risks, and protection. Science, 350(6265), 1193-1198.

[178] Greider, C. W., & Blackburn, E. H. (1985). Identification of a specific telomere terminal transferase activity in Tetrahymena extracts. Cell, 43(2), 405-413.

o Lung cells (pneumocytes)

o Pancreatic cells (pancreatic islet cells)

Somatic cells make up the vast majority of cells in an organism and perform a wide range of functions to support the general health and functioning of the body. They are essential for tissue repair, organ function, and the wellbeing of the organism.

2. **Lifestyle Factors:** Certain lifestyle factors, such as regular exercise, a healthy diet, and stress management, may promote telomere maintenance and lengthening.[179]

3. **Pharmacological Interventions:** Researchers are investigating various compounds and drugs that might enhance telomerase activity or protect telomeres, potentially slowing down the aging process.[180]

Potential Implications for Longevity:

1. **Telomere Length and Longevity:** Some studies suggest that individuals with longer telomeres tend to live longer and have a lower risk of age-related diseases.[181]

2. **Interventions for Healthy Aging:** Telomere lengthening interventions, if proven safe and effective, could offer a promising approach to promoting healthy aging and extending the "health span" of individuals.[182]

---

[179] Ornish, D., Lin, J., Daubenmier, J., Weidner, G., Epel, E., Kemp, C., ... & Blackburn, E. H. (2008). Increased telomerase activity and comprehensive lifestyle changes: A pilot study. The Lancet Oncology, 9(11), 1048-1057.

[180] Jaskelioff, M., Muller, F. L., Paik, J. H., Thomas, E., Jiang, S., Adams, A. C., ... & Depinho, R. A. (2011). Telomerase reactivation reverses tissue degeneration in aged telomerase-deficient mice. Nature, 469(7328), 102-106.

[181] Codd, V., Nelson, C. P., Albrecht, E., Mangino, M., Deelen, J., Buxton, J. L., ... & Samani, N. J. (2013). Identification of seven loci affecting mean telomere length and their association with disease. Nature Genetics, 45(4), 422-427.

[182] Blasco, M. A. (2007). Telomere length, stem cells and aging. Nature Chemical Biology, 3(10), 640-649.

3. **Ethical Considerations:** The use of telomere lengthening interventions for life extension raises ethical questions and requires careful regulation and oversight.[183]

Understanding the role of telomeres in cellular aging and the potential for telomere lengthening interventions is a burgeoning field in longevity research. While many questions remain, the science of telomeres holds promise for advancing our knowledge of aging and age-related diseases.

Strategies for Telomere Lengthening: Extending the Cellular Lifespan

Strategies for telomere lengthening include lifestyle modifications, dietary choices, and emerging therapies like telomerase activation, each with its own potential benefits and limitations in the pursuit of longevity.

Lifestyle Modifications:

A. **Physical Activity:** Regular exercise has been associated with longer telomeres, possibly due to its anti-inflammatory and antioxidant effects.[184]

B. **Stress Reduction:** Managing chronic stress through techniques like meditation and mindfulness may help mitigate telomere shortening by reducing cortisol levels.[185]

---

[183] de Grey, A. D., Ames, B. N., Andersen, J. K., Bartke, A., Campisi, J., Heward, C. B., ... & Sierra, F. (2002). Time to talk SENS: Critiquing the immutability of human aging. Annals of the New York Academy of Sciences, 959(1), 452-462.

[184] Ludlow, A. T., & Roth, S. M. (2011). Physical activity and telomere biology: Exploring the link with aging-related disease prevention. Journal of Aging Research, 2011, 790378.

[185] Epel, E. S., Puterman, E., Lin, J., Blackburn, E. H., & Lum, P. Y. (2013). Meditation and vacation effects have an impact on disease-associated molecular phenotypes. Translational Psychiatry, 3(7), e293.

C. **Sleep Quality:** Poor sleep patterns and insufficient sleep may accelerate telomere attrition, emphasizing the importance of quality sleep for telomere maintenance.[186]

Dietary Choices:

A. **Antioxidant-Rich Diet:** A diet rich in antioxidants from fruits, vegetables, and teas may protect against oxidative stress and support telomere health.[187]

B. **Omega-3 Fatty Acids:** Omega-3 fatty acids, found in fatty fish and flaxseed, have been linked to longer telomeres and reduced cellular aging.[188]

C. **Caloric Restriction:** Caloric restriction, while not fully understood, has shown potential for extending lifespan and maintaining telomere length.[189]

Emerging Therapies:

A. **Telomerase Activation:** Researchers are exploring telomerase activation as a potential therapy to lengthen telomeres. Telomerase gene therapy and small molecules targeting telomerase are under investigation.[190]

---

[186] Prather, A. A., Puterman, E., Lin, J., O'Donovan, A., Krauss, J., Tomiyama, A. J., ... & Epel, E. S. (2011). Shorter leukocyte telomere length in midlife women with poor sleep quality. Journal of Aging Research, 2011, 721390.

[187] Lee, J.Y., Jun, N. R., & Yoon, D. (2017). Association between dietary patterns in the remote past and telomere length. European Journal of Clinical Nutrition, 71(2), 274-279.

[188] Farzaneh-Far, R., Lin, J., Epel, E. S., Harris, W. S., Blackburn, E. H., & Whooley, M. A. (2010). Association of marine omega-3 fatty acid levels with telomeric aging in patients with coronary heart disease. JAMA, 303(3), 250-257.

[189] Vermeulen, M., Klöpping-Ketelaars, I.W., van den Berg, R., Vaes, W. H., & Westerterp, K. R. (2005). Decline in a urinary marker of oxidative stress with ingestion of a solid fat-rich meal is correlated with age in overweight and obese subjects. Free Radical Biology and Medicine, 38(3), 375-381.

[190] Bernardes de Jesus, B., Schneeberger, K., Vera, E., Tejera, A. M., Ayuso, E., Bosch, F., & Blasco, M. A. (2012). Telomerase gene therapy in adult and old mice delays aging and increases longevity without increasing cancer. EMBO Molecular Medicine, 4(8), 691-704.

B. **Senolytics:** Senolytic drugs that selectively remove senescent cells may indirectly support telomere lengthening by removing cells with critically short telomeres.[191]

C. **Gene Editing:** Advances in gene editing technologies, such as CRISPR-Cas9, hold promise for directly modifying telomere length, although ethical and safety considerations remain.[192]

Benefits and Limitations:

1. **Benefits:** Extending telomeres may have potential benefits for delaying age-related diseases and promoting healthy aging, although clinical evidence is still emerging.

2. **Limitations:** The efficacy and safety of many telomere-lengthening strategies, especially emerging therapies, are still under investigation, and long-term effects are unknown.

3. **Ethical Considerations:** Ethical concerns surround the use of certain technologies, such as gene editing, for telomere lengthening and the potential for unintended consequences.[193]

The pursuit of telomere lengthening as a means to extend the cellular lifespan and promote longevity is an exciting area of research. However, caution and careful consideration of the benefits, risks, and ethical implications are essential as this field continues to evolve.

---

[191] Hickson, L. J., Langhi Prata, L. G. P., Bobart, S. A., Evans, T. I Giorgadze, N., Hashmi, S. K., ... & Kirkland, J. L. (2019). Senolytics decrease senescent cells in humans: Preliminary report from a clinical trial of Dasatinib plus Quercetin in individuals with diabetic kidney disease. EBioMedicine, 47, 446-456.

[192] Ocampo, A., Reddy, P., Belmonte, J. C. I., & Antonarakis, S. E. (2016). Gene editing in adult organisms through in vivo somatic cell reprogramming: Are we there yet? Cell Stem Cell, 18(6), 679-680.

[193] Ishii, T. (2014). Germline genome-editing research and its socioethical implications. Trends in Molecular Medicine, 20(7), 375-376.

Supplementation

While there is ongoing research into supplements and compounds that may support telomere length maintenance and potentially enhance telomerase activity, it's important to note that the field is still evolving, and definitive evidence of their efficacy is not yet established. These supplements are not a guarantee of longer telomeres or increased telomerase activity, and their use should be approached with caution. Here are some supplements and compounds that have been studied in relation to telomeres and telomerase:

1. **Astragalus Root (Astragalus membranaceus):** Astragalus is an herb traditionally used in Chinese medicine. Some studies suggest that it may support telomere maintenance and enhance telomerase activity.[194] However, more research is needed to confirm its effects.

2. **TA-65:** TA-65 is a commercial supplement derived from Astragalus that claims to support telomere health. Clinical evidence supporting its effectiveness is limited, and it can be quite expensive.[195]

3. **Fish Oil (Omega-3 Fatty Acids):** Omega-3 fatty acids, found in fish oil supplements, have been associated with longer telomeres in some studies.[196] Omega-3s are known for their anti-inflammatory properties, which may contribute to telomere maintenance.

---

[194] Hofmann, J. N., & Purdue, M. P. (2009). The promise and perils of telomere length measurement for cancer and aging research. Journal of the National Cancer Institute, 101(21), 1457-1459.

[195] Harley, C. B., Liu, W., Blasco, M., Vera, E., & Andrews, W. H. (2011). A natural product telomerase activator as part of a health maintenance program. Rejuvenation Research, 14(1), 45-56.

[196] Farzaneh-Far, R., Lin, J., Epel, E. S., Harris, W. S., Blackburn, E. H., & Whooley, M. A. (2010). Association of marine omega-3 fatty acid levels with telomeric aging in patients with coronary heart disease. JAMA, 303(3), 250-257.

4. **Vitamin D:** Adequate vitamin D levels have been linked to longer telomeres. However, vitamin D supplements should be used cautiously and under the guidance of a healthcare provider, as excessive supplementation can have adverse effects.[197]

5. **Antioxidants:** Antioxidant vitamins such as vitamin C, vitamin E, and coenzyme Q10 have been studied for their potential to protect against oxidative stress, which can contribute to telomere shortening. These vitamins are often found in multivitamin supplements.

6. **Resveratrol:** Found in red wine and certain supplements, resveratrol is being investigated for its potential to activate sirtuins, a group of proteins associated with longevity. However, its effects on telomeres are still unclear.[198]

7. **Curcumin:** Curcumin, a compound found in turmeric, has antioxidant and anti-inflammatory properties. Some research suggests it may positively impact telomere health, but more studies are needed.[199]

8. **N-Acetylcysteine (NAC):** NAC is a supplement that can boost the body's production of glutathione, an antioxidant. It has been studied for its potential to protect against oxidative damage that affects telomeres.[200]

---

[197] Richards, J. B., Valdes, A. M., Gardner, J. P., Paximadas, D., Kimura, M., Nessa, A., ... & Spector, T. D. (2007). Higher serum vitamin D concentrations are associated with longer leukocyte telomere length in women. The American Journal of Clinical Nutrition, 86(5), 1420-1425.

[198] Howitz, K. T., Bitterman, K. J., Cohen, H. Y., Lamming, D. W., Lavu, S., Wood, J. G., ... & Sinclair, D. A. (2003). Small molecule activators of sirtuins extend Saccharomyces cerevisiae lifespan. Nature, 425(6954), 191-196.

[199] Xu, Y., Ku, B. S., Yao, H. Y., Lin, Y. H., Ma, X., Zhang, Y. H., ... & Li, X. J. (2007). The effects of curcumin on depressive-like behaviors in mice. European Journal of Pharmacology, 570(1-3), 77-83.

[200] Al-Nakkash, L., Markus, B., Batia, L., Prozialeck, W. C., & Broderick, T. L. (2008). N-acetylcysteine prevents the decreases in cardiac collagen cross-linking and myocardial stiffness that occur with aging. Journal of Cardiovascular Pharmacology, 52(3), 234-241.

9. **Melatonin:** Melatonin, a hormone that regulates sleep, may have antioxidant properties that protect against telomere shortening associated with poor sleep quality. However, more research is needed.[201]

It's crucial to approach supplementation with caution and consult a healthcare professional before adding any new supplements to your routine, especially if you have underlying health conditions or are taking medications. Furthermore, maintaining a healthy lifestyle, including regular exercise, a balanced diet, stress management, and adequate sleep, remains the foundation for promoting overall health and potentially supporting telomere length and telomerase activity. Remember that the field of telomere biology is still relatively young, and more research is required to fully understand the effects and safety of these supplements on telomeres and aging.

Caloric Restriction and Longevity

The Science of Caloric Restriction: Metabolism, Insulin Sensitivity, and Cellular Repair Mechanisms

Caloric restriction (CR) is a dietary regimen that involves reducing calorie intake while maintaining essential nutrients. It has been studied extensively for its potential health benefits, including effects on metabolism, insulin sensitivity, and cellular repair mechanisms. There are scientific foundations of caloric restriction and its impacts on various aspects of health.

---

[201] Lanoix, D., Guérin, P., Vaillancourt, C., & Melatonin (2012). Melatonin: Drug of choice for human oocyte cryopreservation? Journal of Pineal Research, 53(3), 215-221.

Metabolism and Energy Balance:

1. **Energy Deficit:** Caloric restriction creates an energy deficit, leading to weight loss, which is typically associated with improved metabolic health.[202]

2. **Metabolic Rate:** CR may lead to a decrease in metabolic rate to conserve energy, but this effect tends to be modest and is accompanied by metabolic adaptations.[203]

3. **Mitochondrial Function:** CR can enhance mitochondrial function, improving the efficiency of energy production and reducing oxidative stress.[204]

Insulin Sensitivity and Glucose Regulation:

1. **Improved Insulin Sensitivity:** CR has been shown to enhance insulin sensitivity, reducing the risk of type 2 diabetes and improving glucose regulation.[205]

2. **Reduced Insulin and IGF-1 Levels:** CR lowers circulating insulin and insulin-like growth factor 1 (IGF-1), which are associated with age-related diseases and longevity.[206]

---

[202] Fontana, L., & Klein, S. (2007). Aging, adiposity, and calorie restriction. JAMA, 297(9), 986-994.

[203] Ravussin, E., Redman, L. M., RocholJ., Das, S. K., Fontana, L., Kraus, W. E., ... & the CALERIE Study Group. (2015). A 2-year randomized controlled trial of human caloric restriction: Feasibility and effects on predictors of health span and longevity. Journals of Gerontology Series A: Biomedical Sciences and Medical Sciences, 70(9), 1097-1104.

[204] López-Lluch, G., Hunt, N., Jones, B., Zhu, M., Jamieson, H., Hilmer, S., ... & de Cabo, R. (2006). Calorie restriction induces mitochondrial biogenesis and bioenergetic efficiency. Proceedings of the National Academy of Sciences, 103(6), 1768-1773.

[205] Larson-Meyer, D. E., Heilbronn, L. K., Redman, L.I, Newcomer, B. R., Frisard, M. I., Anton, S., ... & Ravussin, E. (2006). Effect of calorie restriction with or without exercise on insulin sensitivity, beta-cell function, fat cell size, and ectopic lipid in overweight subjects. Diabetes Care, 29(6), 1337-1344.

[206] Fontana, L., Weiss, E. P., Villareal, D.T., Klein, S., & Holloszy, J. O. (2008). Long-term effects of calorie or protein restriction on serum IGF-1 and IGFBP-3 concentration in humans. Aging Cell, 7(5), 681-687.

3. **Enhanced Beta-Cell Function:** CR can preserve beta-cell function in the pancreas, which is crucial for insulin production.[207]

Cellular Repair Mechanisms:

1. **Autophagy:** Caloric restriction promotes autophagy, a cellular process that removes damaged components and supports cellular repair and longevity.[208]

2. **Sirtuins:** CR activates sirtuins, a family of proteins associated with longevity and the regulation of cellular processes such as DNA repair and gene expression.[209]

3. **DNA Repair:** CR may enhance DNA repair mechanisms, reducing the accumulation of DNA damage associated with aging.[210]

Longevity and Health Span:

1. **Extended Lifespan:** Studies in various organisms, including mice and primates, have demonstrated that CR can extend lifespan and delay the onset of age-related diseases.[211]

---

[207] Shinmura, K., Tamaki, K., Saito, K., Nakano, Y., Tobe, T., & Bolli, R. Cardioprotective Effects of Short-Term Caloric Restriction Are Mediated by Adiponectin via Activation of AMP-Activated Protein Kinase. Circulation, 116(24), 2809-2817.

[208] Madeo, F., Pietrocola, F., Eisenberg, T., & Kroemer, G. (2018). Caloric restriction mimetics: Toward a molecular definition. Nature Reviews Drug Discovery, 17(12), 889-904.

[209] Guarente, L. (2013). Calorie restriction and sirtuins revisited. Genes & Development, 27(19), 2072-2085.

[210] Lombard, D. B., Chua, K. F., Mostoslavsky, R., Franco, S., Gostissa, M., Alt, F.W., & Guarente, L. (2005). DNA repair, genome stability, and aging. Cell, 120(4), 497-512.

[211] Mattison, J. A., Colman, R. J., Beasley, IM., Allison, D. B., Kemnitz, J. W., Roth, G. S., ... & Anderson, R. M. (2017). Caloric restriction improves health and survival of rhesus monkeys. Nature Communications, 8, 14063.

2. **Health Span:** While CR may not be feasible for long-term human use, its potential to extend health span by reducing the risk of age-related diseases is of significant interest.[212]

3. **Intermittent Fasting:** Intermittent fasting, a less extreme form of caloric restriction, is also being investigated for its potential health benefits, including improved metabolism and longevity.[213]

Caloric restriction is a complex dietary strategy with significant effects on metabolism, insulin sensitivity, and cellular repair mechanisms. While research in animals has shown promising results, the translation of CR's benefits to human health requires further investigation and consideration of the practicality and sustainability of such dietary approaches.

The Science of Fasting and Intermittent Fasting (IF): Autophagy, Cellular Rejuvenation, and Potential Longevity

Fasting and intermittent fasting are biohacking strategies that mimic the effects of caloric restriction. These practices, including autophagy, cellular rejuvenation, and potential longevity, have real benefits when incorporated into an anti-aging regimen.

Autophagy:

A. **Cellular Cleaning:** Fasting induces autophagy, a process where cells remove damaged or dysfunctional components, contributing to cellular health and longevity.[214]

---

[212] Fontana, L., & Partridge, L. (2015). Promoting health and longevity through diet: From model organisms to humans. Cell, 161(1), 106-118.

[213] Longo, V. D., & Mattson, M. P. (2014). Fasting: Molecular mechanisms and clinical applications. Cell Metabolism, 19(2), 181-192.

[214] Mizushima, N., & Komatsu, M. (2011). Autophagy: Renovation of cells and tissues. Cell, 147(4), 728-741.

B. **Clearing Protein Aggregates:** Autophagy helps clear protein aggregates associated with neurodegenerative diseases, potentially reducing the risk of such conditions.[215]

C. **Improved Cellular Function:** By recycling cellular components, autophagy can rejuvenate cells, leading to improved cellular function and resilience.[216]

Cellular Rejuvenation:

A. **Stem Cell Regeneration:** Fasting may stimulate the regeneration of stem cells, contributing to tissue repair and rejuvenation.[217]

B. **Enhanced Mitochondrial Function:** Fasting can enhance mitochondrial function, improving energy production and reducing oxidative stress.[218]

C. **Inflammation Reduction:** Fasting can reduce chronic inflammation, a key driver of age-related diseases.[219]

Longevity:

A. **Animal Studies:** Studies in model organisms like yeast, worms, flies, and mice have shown that fasting can extend lifespan and improve health span.[220]

---

[215] Rubinsztein, D. C., Mariño, G., & Kroemer, G. (2011). Autophagy and aging. Cell, 146(5), 682-695.

[216] Madeo, F., Pietrocola, F., Eisenberg, T., & Kroemer, G. (2018). Caloric restriction mimetics: Towards a molecular definition. Nature Reviews Drug Discovery, 17(12), 889-904.

[217] Cheng, C. W., AIs, G. B., Perin, L., Wei, M., Zhou, X., Lam, B. S., ... & Longo, V. D. (2014). Prolonged fasting reduces IGF-1/PKA to promote hematopoietic-stem-cell-based regeneration and reverse immunosuppression. Cell Stem Cell, 14(6), 810-823.

[218] Brandhorst, S., Choi, I.I, Wei, M., Cheng, C. W., Sedrakyan, S., Navarrete, G., ... & Longo, V. D. (2015). A periodic diet that mimics fasting promotes multi-system regeneration, enhanced cognitive performance, and healthspan. Cell Metabolism, 22(1), 86-99.

[219] SafdieI., Brandhorst, S., Wei, M., Wang, W., Lee, C., Hwang, S., ... & Longo, V. D. (2012). Fasting enhances the response of glioma to chemo- and radiotherapy. PLoS One, 7(9), e44603.

[220] Longo, V. D., & Mattson, M. P. (2014). Fasting: Molecular mechanisms and clinical applications. Cell Metabolism, 19(2), 181-192.

B. **Human Studies:** While human research is ongoing, some studies suggest that intermittent fasting and calorie restriction mimetics may have longevity benefits.[221]

Fasting Protocols:

A. **Intermittent Fasting (IF):** IF involves cycles of eating and fasting, with popular methods like the 16/8 (16 hours of fasting, 8 hours of eating) and the 5:2 diet (eating normally for 5 days and restricting calories for 2 days).[222]

B. **Time-Restricted Eating (TRE):** TRE limits daily eating to a specific time window, such as 8 hours, promoting overnight fasting.[223]

C. **Periodic Fasting:** Longer fasts, such as alternate-day fasting or multi-day water fasts, can induce more profound autophagy and cellular rejuvenation.[224]

Incorporating Fasting into Anti-Aging Regimens:

A. **Consultation:** Before beginning any fasting regimen, individuals should consult with a healthcare provider, especially if they have underlying health conditions or are taking medications.

B. **Gradual Transition:** Gradually introduce fasting protocols to allow the body to adapt.

---

[221] Anton, S. D., Moel K., Donahoo, W. T., Marosi, K., Lee, S. A., Mainous, A. G., ... & Mattson, M. P. (2018). Flipping the metabolic switch: Understanding and applying the health benefits of fasting. Obesity, 26(2), 254-268.

[222] Patterson, R. E., Laughlin, G.I, LaCroix, A. Z., Hartman, S. J., Natarajan, L., Senger, C. M., ... & Villasante, U. (2015). Intermittent fasting and human metabolic health. JAMA Internal Medicine, 175(5), 734-743.

[223] Wilkinson, M. J., Manoogian, E. N., Zadourian, A., Lo, H., Fakhouri, S., Shoghi, A., ... & Panda, S. (2020). Ten-hour time-restricted eating reduces weight, blood pressure, and atherogenic lipids in patients with metabolic syndrome. Cell Metabolism, 31(1), 92-104.

[224] Mattson, M. P., Longo, V. D., & Harvie, M. (2017). Impact of intermittent fasting on health and disease processes. Ageing Research Reviews, 39, 46-58.

C. **Hydration and Nutrition:** Stay well-hydrated during fasting periods and prioritize nutrient-dense foods during eating windows.

D. **Monitoring:** Consider monitoring biomarkers and seeking regular health check-ups when incorporating fasting into an anti-aging regimen.

Fasting, when approached mindfully and responsibly, can be a valuable component of an anti-aging regimen. However, individual responses to fasting can vary. As such, more research is needed to fully understand its long-term effects on human health and aging.

Cutting-Edge Anti-Aging Therapies

Innovative Approaches in Anti-Aging: Senolytics, NAD+ Supplementation, Gene Therapy, and Stem Cells

Anti-aging science continues to evolve, leading to the development of cutting-edge therapies that challenge the boundaries of the human lifespan. Innovative approaches such as senolytics, NAD+ supplementation, gene therapy, and the use of stem cells help us discover the promise and potential risks associated with these groundbreaking therapies.

Senolytics: Unleashing the Power of Youthful Cells

"Senolytics" refers to a class of drugs or compounds that are being developed and studied for their potential to selectively target and eliminate senescent cells from the body. Senescent cells are cells that have entered a state of irreversible growth arrest, typically as a response to stress, DNA damage, or aging. While senescent cells play a role in wound healing and tissue repair, the accumulation of senescent cells over time is associated with aging and age-related diseases.

These compounds are designed to selectively target and remove senescent cells—cells that have ceased to divide and contribute to the aging process. The idea is to clear these aging cells to rejuvenate our tissues and potentially extend our lifespan.[225] Early studies in animals have shown that senolytics can enhance tissue function, reduce inflammation, and bolster overall health.[226] While clinical trials are ongoing to evaluate their safety and effectiveness in humans, the field is rife with excitement and potential.[227]

NAD+ Supplementation: Fueling Cellular Vitality

Nicotinamide adenine dinucleotide (NAD+) is a coenzyme that plays a critical role in cellular energy production and DNA repair. Unfortunately, NAD+ levels decline with age, leading to cellular dysfunction. Researchers are exploring NAD+ supplementation as a way to reverse this decline. Compounds like nicotinamide riboside (NR) and nicotinamide mononucleotide (NMN) show promise as NAD+ boosters, potentially supporting mitochondrial function, DNA repair, and sirtuin activity—all factors linked to longevity.[228]

Dr. David Sinclair, a renowned biologist and professor, is well-known for his research into the role of NAD+ in aging and longevity.

---

[225] Kirkland, J. L., & Tchkonia, T. (2017). Cellular senescence: A translational perspective. EBioMedicine, 21, 21-28.

[226] Justice, J. N., Niedernhofer, L., Robbins, P. D., & Schafer, M. J. (2019). Senolytics in idiopathic pulmonary fibrosis: Results from a first-in-human, open-label, pilot study. EBioMedicine, 40, 554-563.

[227] Hickson, L. J., Langhi Prata, L. G. P., Bobart, S. A., Evans, T. K., Giorgadze, N., Hashmi, S. K., ... & Kirkland, J. L. (2019). Senolytics decrease senescent cells in humans: Preliminary report from a clinical trial of Dasatinib plus Quercetin in individuals with diabetic kidney disease. EBioMedicine, 47, 446-456.

[228] Verdin, E. (2015). NAD+ in aging, metabolism, and neurodegeneration. Science, 350(6265), 1208-1213; Trammell, S. A., Schmidt, M. S., Weidemann, B. J., Redpath, P., Jaksch, F., Dellinger, R. W., ... & Brenner, C. (2016). Nicotinamide riboside is uniquely and orally bioavailable in mice and humans. Nature Communications, 7, 12948; Mouchiroud, L., Houtkooper, R. H., Moullan, N., Katsyuba, E., Ryu, D., Cantó, C., ... & Auwerx, J. (2013). The NAD+/sirtuin pathway modulates longevity through activation of mitochondrial UPR and FOXO signaling. Cell, 154(2), 430-441.

NAD+ has been a central focus of his work, and his research has contributed significantly to our understanding of how NAD+ levels can influence various biological processes.

Here are key aspects of Dr. David Sinclair's work related to NAD+:

A. **NAD+ Depletion and Aging:** Dr. Sinclair's research has highlighted the link between declining NAD+ levels and the aging process. NAD+ is involved in many critical cellular processes, and its levels tend to decrease with age. This decline is thought to contribute to cellular dysfunction and age-related health issues.

B. **NAD+ Precursors:** Dr. Sinclair's work has explored the use of NAD+ precursors, such as nicotinamide mononucleotide (NMN) and nicotinamide riboside (NR), as potential interventions to boost NAD+ levels. These precursors can be converted into NAD+ in the body and may help counteract the effects of NAD+ decline associated with aging.

C. **Sirtuins:** Dr. Sinclair's research has focused on sirtuins, a family of enzymes that require NAD+ as a cofactor. Sirtuins play critical roles in regulating gene expression, DNA repair, and various cellular processes. Dr. Sinclair has investigated how NAD+ supplementation can activate sirtuins and potentially enhance cellular health and longevity.

D. **Health Benefits:** While much of Dr. Sinclair's work has been conducted on animal models, it has sparked interest in the potential health benefits of NAD+ supplementation for humans. Some of the proposed benefits include improved mitochondrial function, enhanced DNA repair, and potentially extending health span.

E. **Clinical Trials:** Dr. Sinclair has been involved in clinical trials investigating the safety and efficacy of NAD+ precursors in humans. These trials aim to determine whether NAD+ supplementation can have positive effects on age-related conditions and overall health.

It's important to note that while the research on NAD+ and its potential benefits is promising, it is still an evolving field, and further studies are needed to fully understand the long-term effects and safety of NAD+ supplementation in humans. Additionally, Dr. Sinclair's work has sparked broader interest in the field of aging biology and has contributed to ongoing research into interventions that may slow down the aging process and improve health in later years.[229]

Gene Therapy: Rewriting the Blueprint of Aging

Advances in gene editing technologies, most notably CRISPR–Cas9, are revolutionizing the possibilities for modifying genes associated with aging and age-related diseases. Gene therapy opens up exciting

---

[229] Sinclair, D. A., & Guarente, L. (1997). Extrachromosomal rDNA circles--a cause of aging in yeast. Cell, 91(7), 1033-1042. This is one of Dr. Sinclair's early research papers on aging-related mechanisms in yeast cells; Imai, S., Armstrong, C. M., Kaeberlein, M., & Guarente, L. (2000). Transcriptional silencing and longevity protein Sir2 is an NAD-dependent histone deacetylase. Nature, 403(6771), 795-800. This paper discusses the role of Sir2 (a sirtuin) and NAD+ in gene regulation and longevity in yeast, laying the groundwork for subsequent research in the field; Imai, S., & Guarente, L. (2014). NAD+ and sirtuins in aging and disease. Trends in Cell Biology, 24(8), 464-471. This review article by Dr. Sinclair and Dr. Leonard Guarente provides an overview of the connection between NAD+, sirtuins, and aging; Bonkowski, M. S., & Sinclair, D. A. (2016). Slowing ageing by design: The rise of NAD+ and sirtuin-activating compounds. Nature Reviews Molecular Cell Biology, 17(11), 679-690. This review discusses the potential of NAD+ and sirtuin-activating compounds as interventions to slow down aging; Yoshino, J., Baur, J. A., & Imai, S. (2018). NAD+ intermediates: The biology and therapeutic potential of NMN and NR. Cell Metabolism, 27(3), 513-528. This paper explores the use of NAD+ precursors, including NMN and NR, and their potential benefits for health and longevity. Rajman, L., Chwalek, K., & Sinclair, D. A. (2018). Therapeutic potential of NAD-boosting molecules: The in vivo evidence. Cell Metabolism, 27(3), 529-547. This review discusses the in vivo evidence and potential therapeutic applications of NAD-boosting molecules; Tony Robbins, Peter Diamandis & Robert Hariri (2022). Life Force. Simon & Schuster. 95-120.

prospects for intervening at the genetic level to combat the aging process.[230] For instance, telomerase gene therapy strives to extend telomeres, the protective caps on our chromosomes that tend to shorten with age, potentially slowing cellular aging.[231] However, ethical concerns and rigorous safety considerations are paramount in gene therapy research.[232]

Stem Cells: The Regenerative Powerhouses

Stem cells have long held promise for their regenerative potential. Stem cell therapies seek to harness this power to repair damaged tissues and organs, offering the tantalizing prospect of rejuvenation.[233] Induced pluripotent stem cells (iPSCs), in particular, enable the generation of patient-specific cells for transplantation and tissue repair, a promising avenue for personalized medicine.[234] Yet, the field grapples with the challenges of ensuring safety and efficacy while navigating ethical considerations.[235]

---

[230] Doudna, J. A., & Charpentier, E. (2014). Genome editing. The new frontier of genome engineering with CRISPR-Cas9. Science, 346(6213), 1258096.

[231] Bernardes de Jesus, B., Schneeberger, K., Vera, E., Tejera, A. M., Ayuso, E., Bosch, F., & Blasco, M. A. (2012). Telomerase gene therapy in adult and old mice.

[232] Gyngell, C., Douglas, T., & Savulescu, J. (2019). The ethics of germline gene editing. Journal of Applied Philosophy, 36(1), 5-24. This article explores the ethical considerations surrounding germline gene editing, a specific area of gene therapy research that involves making heritable changes to an individual's genome. It emphasizes the need for ethical reflection and robust safety measures in gene editing technologies.

[233] Imai, S., Armstrong, C. M., Kaeberlein, M., & Guarente, L. (2000). Transcriptional silencing and longevity protein Sir2 is an NAD-dependent histone deacetylase. Nature, 403(6771), 795-800. This paper discusses the role of Sir2 (a sirtuin) and NAD+ in gene regulation and longevity in yeast, laying the groundwork for subsequent research in the field.

[234] Imai, S., & Guarente, L. (2014). NAD+ and sirtuins in aging and disease. Trends in Cell Biology, 24(8), 464-471. This review article by Dr. Sinclair and Dr. Leonard Guarente provides an overview of the connection between NAD+, sirtuins, and aging.

[235] Bonkowski, M. S., & Sinclair, D. A. (2016). Slowing ageing by design: The rise of NAD+ and sirtuin-activating compounds. Nature Reviews Molecular Cell Biology, 17(11), 679-690. This review discusses the potential of NAD+ and sirtuin-activating compounds as interventions to slow down aging.

Balancing Promise and Prudence

These innovative approaches in anti-aging science offer the potential to rejuvenate tissues, delay age-related diseases, and extend health span. However, they also come with their share of risks and uncertainties. Safety and ethical considerations are pivotal, and ongoing research is crucial to understand the full spectrum of benefits and potential drawbacks.[236] Personalized medicine, tailoring these therapies to individual needs and genetic profiles, is an important aspect of their development and application.

As we venture into these uncharted territories of anti-aging science, we must balance the promise of a longer, healthier life with the wisdom of responsible and ethical research. The future of aging is an exciting frontier where science and prudence walk hand in hand.

Personalized Anti-Aging Strategies

Biohackers understand that there is no one-size-fits-all approach to anti-aging. Factors including genetics, lifestyle, and individual goals are key to optimizing individualized results.

Personalized Anti-Aging Strategies: Unlocking Your Unique Path to Youthful Aging

Every individual is unique, with a distinct genetic makeup, lifestyle, and personal goals. The crucial importance of personalized anti-aging strategies cannot be emphasized enough. Exploring insights into how to tailor an anti-aging regimen to achieve optimal results, considering specific genetic factors, lifestyle choices, and individual objectives are key.

---

[236] Yoshino, J., Baur, J. A., & Imai, S. (2018). NAD+ intermediates: The biology and therapeutic potential of NMN and NR. Cell Metabolism, 27(3), 513-528. This paper explores the use of NAD+ precursors, including NMN and NR, and their potential benefits for health and longevity. Rajman, L., Chwalek, K., & Sinclair, D. A. (2018). Therapeutic potential of NAD-boosting molecules: The in vivo evidence. Cell Metabolism, 27(3), 529-547. This review discusses the in vivo evidence and potential therapeutic applications of NAD-boosting molecules.

Genetic Variability: The Blueprint of Aging

1. **Understanding Genetic Factors:** Genetics play a significant role in determining how we age. Some individuals may be genetically predisposed to certain age-related conditions, while others possess genetic variants associated with longevity.[237]

2. **Genetic Testing:** Genetic testing and analysis can provide valuable insights into your genetic profile, allowing for the identification of specific genetic markers related to aging and disease risk.[238]

3. **Personalized Risk Assessment:** Armed with genetic information, you can work with healthcare professionals to create a personalized risk assessment for age-related conditions and tailor preventive measures accordingly.[239]

Lifestyle Choices: Nurturing Your Wellbeing

1. **Dietary References:** Personalized anti-aging strategies take into account your dietary preferences, whether you lean toward Mediterranean, plant-based, ketogenic, or other dietary patterns.[240]

2. **Exercise Regimens:** Tailored fitness plans consider your fitness level, preferences, and goals, whether it's endurance, strength training, yoga, or a combination.[241]

---

[237] López-Otín, C., Blasco, M.A., Partridge, L., Serrano, M., & Kroemer, G. (2013). The hallmarks of aging. Cell, 153(6), 1194-1217.

[238] Caulfield, T., & Murdoch, B. (2017). Genes, cells, and biobanks: Yes, there's still a consent problem. PLOS Biology, 15(7), e2002654.

[239] Nielson, C. M., & Klein, R. F. (2019). Viewpoint: Personalized medicine for osteoporosis: Closer to reality. The Journal of Clinical Endocrinology & Metabolism, 104(10), 4378-4386.

[240] Grosso, G., Micek, A., Marventano, S., Castellano, S., & Galvano, F. (2015). Dietary n-3 PUFA, fish consumption and depression: A systematic review and meta-analysis of observational studies. Journal of Affective Disorders, 205, 269-281.

[241] Kraemer, W. J., & Ratamess, N. A. (2004). Fundamentals of resistance training: Progression and exercise prescription. Medicine & Science in Sports & Exercise, 36(4), 674-688.

3. **Sleep Optimization:** Recognizing the importance of sleep hygiene and understanding your unique sleep patterns is vital for creating a personalized anti-aging plan.[242]

4. **Stress Management:** Lifestyle choices encompass stress management techniques, such as meditation, mindfulness, or other relaxation practices that resonate with you.[243]

Individual Objectives: Defining Your Path

1. **Defining Priorities:** Personalized anti-aging strategies allow individuals to define their priorities, whether it's optimizing physical performance, preserving cognitive function, or addressing specific health concerns.[244]

2. **Setting Realistic Goals:** Personalized plans involve setting realistic and achievable goals, taking into account an individual's current health status and long-term aspirations.[245]

• **Monitoring and Adjustments:** Regular monitoring of progress and making adjustments based on individual responses are key to the success of personalized anti-aging strategies.[246]

Consultation and Collaboration: The Role of Experts

1. **Healthcare Professionals:** Consulting with healthcare professionals, including genetic counselors, dietitians, fitness

---

[242] Walker, M. P. (2017). Why We Sleep: Unlocking the Power of Sleep and Dreams. Simon and Schuster.

[243] Chiesa, A., & Serretti, A. (2009). Mindfulness-based stress reduction for stress management in healthy people: A review and meta-analysis. The Journal of Alternative and Complementary Medicine, 15(5), 593-600.

[244] Luyten, P., & Blatt, S. J. (2013). Interpersonal relatedness and self-definition in normal and disrupted personality development: Retrospect and prospect. American Psychologist, 68(3), 172-183.

[245] Locke, E. A., & Latham, G. P. (2006). New directions in goal-setting theory. Current Directions in Psychological Science, 15(5), 265-268.

[246] Hall, E. E., Ekkekakis, P., & Petruzzello, S. J. (2002). The affective beneficence of vigorous exercise revisited. British Journal of Health Psychology, 7(1), 47-66.

trainers, and physicians, can help individuals create and implement personalized anti-aging plans.[247]

2. **Collaborative Approach:** Building a collaborative relationship with healthcare experts ensures that anti-aging strategies are evidence-based and aligned with individual health needs.[248]

3. **Adaptive Plans:** Personalized strategies are adaptive, allowing for modifications as an individual's goals or health status evolve over time.[249]

Personalized anti-aging strategies are the key to unlocking the full potential of one's journey toward youthful aging. By considering genetic factors, lifestyle choices, and individual objectives, individuals can chart a path that is uniquely tailored to their needs and aspirations. Embracing the diversity of human aging and recognizing the importance of a personalized approach are the cornerstone of a successful anti-aging regimen.

The pursuit of longevity and anti-aging is a dynamic journey that combines scientific understanding with innovative interventions. By unraveling the science of aging and exploring the options set forth in this chapter, you can take proactive steps to extend your health span and lead vibrant, fulfilling lives.

---

[247] Bauer, U. E., Briss, P. A., Goodman, R. A., & Bowman, B. A. (2014). Prevention of chronic disease in the 21st century: Elimination of the leading preventable causes of premature death and disability in the USA. The Lancet, 384(9937), 45-52.

[248] Topol, E. J. (2015). The Patient Will See You Now: The Future of Medicine Is in Your Hands. Basic Books.

[249] Provost, L. P., Murray, S. K., & The Health Care Delivery Subcommittee of the Health Level 7 Clinical Decision Support Work Group. (2014). The Health Care Data Guide: Learning from Data for Improvement. John Wiley & Sons.

CHAPTER 8

BIOHACKING YOUR ENVIRONMENT

Optimizing Health and Sustainability

Your environment plays a pivotal role in shaping your health and wellbeing. In this chapter, we explore the profound influence of your surroundings on your physical and mental health. We'll dive into the art of detoxification, minimizing exposure to environmental toxins, protecting yourself from electromagnetic fields (EMF), optimizing your home for wellbeing, and biohacking for a sustainable future.

Environment and Wellbeing: Nurturing Health Through Surroundings

The Wellness Oasis

Your environment is more than just a backdrop to your life; it's a dynamic force that shapes your health. This section examines how your surroundings impact your physical and mental wellbeing. From air quality and natural light to the layout of your living space, the intricate connections between your environment and your health must be examined.

Air Quality: Breathing Freshness into Life

A. **Indoor Air Pollution:** Poor indoor air quality can lead to various health issues, including respiratory problems, allergies, and decreased cognitive function.[250]

B. **Ventilation and Filtration:** Proper ventilation and air filtration systems help remove pollutants, ensuring a healthier indoor environment.[251]

C. **Natural Air Purifiers:** Houseplants can act as natural air purifiers, enhancing air quality and fostering a sense of wellbeing.[252]

Natural Light: Illuminating Health

A. **Circadian Rhythms:** Exposure to natural light regulates circadian rhythms, influencing sleep patterns, mood, and overall health.[253]

B. **Vitamin D Production:** Sunlight is a natural source of vitamin D, essential for bone health and immune function.[254]

C. **Enhancing Productivity:** Well-lit workspaces improve productivity and reduce the risk of eye strain and fatigue.[255]

---

[250] Sundell, J. (2004). On the history of indoor air quality and health. Indoor Air, 14(s7), 51-58.

[251] Persily, A. K. (2017). Challenges in IAQ measurement and interpretation. Indoor Air, 27(1), 3-7.

[252] Wolverton, B. C., Johnson, A., & Bounds, K. (1989). Interior landscape plants for indoor air pollution abatement. NASA.

[253] Figueiro, M. G., & Rea, M. S. (2010). The effects of red and blue lights on circadian variations in cortisol, alpha amylase, and melatonin. International Journal of Endocrinology.

[254] Holick, M. F. (2007). Vitamin D deficiency. New England Journal of Medicine, 357(3), 266-281.

[255] Heschong, L. (2003). Windows and offices: A study of office worker performance and the indoor environment (No. LBNL-51856).

Layout and Organization: Harmony in Design

A. **Clutter and Stress:** A cluttered living space can lead to increased stress and decreased focus.[256]

B. **Functional Design:** An organized and functional layout supports daily routines and promotes a sense of control.[257]

C. **Biophilic Design:** Incorporating elements of nature, such as natural materials and views of green spaces, has been shown to reduce stress and enhance wellbeing.[258]

Sound Environment: The Power of Acoustics

A. **Noise Pollution:** Chronic exposure to noise pollution can lead to stress, sleep disturbances, and adverse health effects.[259]

B. **Soundscaping:** Thoughtful soundscaping, such as using soothing sounds or white noise, can create a calming environment.[260]

Color Psychology: Painting Emotions

A. **Color Influence:** Colors have psychological effects on mood and behavior. Warm colors can evoke energy, while cool colors promote relaxation.[261]

---

[256] Saxbe, D. E., Repetti, R. L., & Graesch, A. P. (2011). Time spent in home management predicts reduced fat intake among partnered women. The Annals of Behavioral Medicine, 42(3), 405-411.

[257] Carrothers, R. M., & Gregory, W. L. (2008). A review of the literature on the impact of the physical office environment on motivation, performance, and wellbeing. Facilities, 26(3/4), 138-155.

[258] Beatley, T. (2011). Biophilic Cities: Integrating Nature into Urban Design and Planning. Island Press.

[259] Stansfeld, S., & Matheson, M. (2003). Noise pollution: Non-auditory effects on health. British Medical Bulletin, 68(1), 243-257.

[260] Park, J., & Chung, H. (2016). Soundscape and noise control in the urban environment: A review. Applied Sciences, 6(11), 338.

[261] Kwallek, N., Woodson, H., Lewis, C. M., & Sales, C. (1997). Impact of three interior color schemes on worker mood and performance relative to individual environmental sensitivity. Color Research & Application, 22(2), 121-132.

 B. **Personal Preferences:** Consider individual color preferences to create a personalized and emotionally supportive environment.[262]

Green Spaces: Nature's Healing Touch

 A. **Biophilia:** Spending time in green spaces and natural environments has been linked to reduced stress, improved mood, and enhanced mental wellbeing.[263]

 B. **Urban Planning:** Access to parks and green urban planning can positively impact physical health and community wellbeing.[264]

Environmental Consciousness: Sustainable Living

 A. **Eco-Friendly Living:** Sustainable practices, such as reducing waste and conserving resources, contribute to a healthier planet and a sense of purpose.[265]

 B. **Holistic Wellness:** Environmental wellbeing is interconnected with personal wellbeing, emphasizing the importance of sustainability.[266]

Your environment is not just a backdrop to your life; it's a vital component that can either enhance or hinder your physical and mental health. By understanding and optimizing your surroundings,

[262] Ou, L. C., Luo, M. R., Woodcock, A., & Wright, A. (2004). A study of colour emotion and colour preference. Part I: Colour emotions for single colours. Color Research & Application, 29(3), 232-240.

[263] Bratman, G. N., Hamilton, J. P., & Daily, G. C. (2012). The impacts of nature experience on human cognitive function and mental health. Annals of the New York Academy of Sciences, 1249(1), 118-136.

[264] Kaczynski, A. T., & Henderson, K. A. (2007). Environmental correlates of physical activity: A review of evidence about parks and recreation. Leisure Sciences, 29(4), 315-354.

[265] Steg, L., & Vlek, C. (2009). Encouraging pro-environmental behaviour: An integrative review and research agenda. Journal of Environmental Psychology, 29(3), 309-317.

[266] PrilleltenskII., Dietz, S., Prilleltensky, O., Myers, N. D., Rubenstein, C. L., Jin, Y., ... & McMahon, A. (2015). Assessing multidimensional wellbeing: Development and validation of the I COPPE scale. Journal of Community Psychology, 43(2), 199-226.

you can cultivate a space that nurtures your wellbeing and supports a healthier, happier life.

Biophilia: The Healing Bond Between Humans and Nature

Nature is a powerful healer. We introduce the concept of biophilia and how connecting with the natural world can improve your mood, reduce stress, and boost creativity. Biohackers understand the importance of integrating nature into their daily lives, whether through houseplants, outdoor activities, or green spaces.

Biophilia: Nature's Embrace

A. **Evolutionary Roots:** Biophilia suggests that our deep connection with nature has evolutionary roots, as our ancestors relied on the natural world for survival.[267]

B. **Restorative Power:** Nature offers a restorative effect on the human mind and body, promoting relaxation and reducing stress.[268]

C. **Enhanced Creativity:** Exposure to natural environments can enhance creativity and problem-solving abilities, fostering innovative thinking.[269]

Biophilic Design: Bringing Nature Indoors

A. **Indoor Plants:** Houseplants not only improve indoor air quality but also provide a calming and aesthetic connection to nature.[270]

---

[267] Wilson, E. O. (1984). Biophilia. Harvard University Press.

[268] Kaplan, R., & Kaplan, S. (1989). The Experience of Nature: A Psychological Perspective. Cambridge University Press.

[269] Atchley, R. A., Strayer, D. L., & Atchley, P. (2012). Creativity in the wild: Improving creative reasoning through immersion in natural settings. PLoS ONE, 7(12), e51474.

[270] Lohr, V. I., Pearson-Mims, C. H., & Goodwin, G. K. (1996). Interior plants may improve worker productivity and reduce stress in a windowless environment. Journal of Environmental Horticulture, 14(2), 97-100.

B. **Natural Materials:** Incorporating natural materials like wood, stone, and natural textiles into interior design can create a soothing environment.[271]

C. **Views of Nature:** Access to outdoor views or nature-inspired artwork can have positive effects on wellbeing.[272]

Nature's Therapeutic Benefits: A Biohacker's Ally

A. **Forest Bathing:** Shinrin-Yoku, or forest bathing, involves immersing oneself in the forest to reduce stress and boost immune function.[273]

B. **Green Exercise:** Physical activities in natural settings, such as hiking, cycling, or running, combine the benefits of exercise with the healing power of nature.[274]

C. **Mindful Connection:** Mindfulness practices in natural settings promote stress reduction and mental clarity.[275]

Urban Biophilia: Creating Green Spaces

A. **Green Urban Planning:** Biohackers living in urban environments advocate for green urban planning, which includes parks, green roofs, and community gardens.[276]

[271] Ryan, C. O., Browning, W. D., & Clancy, J. O. (2014). Biophilic design patterns: Emerging nature-based parameters for health and wellbeing in the built environment. Environmental Science & Technology, 48(24), 12476-12486.

[272] Tennessen, C. M., & Cimprich, B. (1995). Views to nature: Effects on attention. Journal of Environmental Psychology, 15(1), 77-85.

[273] Li, Q. (2010). Effect of forest bathing trips on human immune function. Environmental Health and Preventive Medicine, 15(1), 9-17.

[274] Pretty, J., Peacock, J., Hine, R., Sellens, M., South, N., & Griffin, M. (2007). Green exercise in the UK countryside: Effects on health and psychological wellbeing, and implications for policy and planning. Journal of Environmental Planning and Management, 50(2), 211-231.

[275] Jordan, M., Hinds, J., & Mackay, G. (2016). Mindfulness for outdoor leadership. Journal of Experiential Education, 39(1), 78-92.

[276] Kuo, F. E., & Sullivan, W. C. (2001). Environment and crime in the inner city: Does vegetation reduce crime? Environment and Behavior, 33(3), 343-367.

B. **Community Engagement:** Involvement in urban gardening and conservation projects fosters a sense of community and wellbeing.[277]

C. **Biophilic Architecture:** Incorporating green elements into city architecture, such as vertical gardens or green facades, brings nature to urban dwellers.[278]

The Biohacker's Connection: Integrating Nature

A. **Daily Rituals:** Biohackers prioritize daily rituals that involve nature, such as morning walks, outdoor meditation, or tending to houseplants.

B. **Tech-Free Nature:** Disconnecting from screens and spending time in natural environments without digital distractions enhances the biophilic experience.[279]

C. **Nature Retreats:** Periodic retreats to natural settings allow biohackers to recharge, refocus, and reconnect with their biophilic instincts.[280]

Understanding and embracing the concept of biophilia can be a transformative part of a biohacker's journey. By nurturing a deeper connection with nature, biohackers harness its therapeutic benefits to optimize their overall wellbeing.

---

[277] Alaimo, K., Beavers, A. W., Crawford, C., Snyder, E. H., & Litt, J. S. Amplifying Community-Based Participatory Research (CBPR) Coalition. (2010). Amplifying community voices to shape public policy at the city level: A case study of the Healthy Neighborhoods Oakland Project. Family & Community Health, 33(1), 26-34.

[278] Brown, G., & Gifford, R. (2001). Architects' views of nature and city life: A cross-cultural comparison. Journal of Environmental Psychology, 21(1), 15-27.

[279] Hartig, T., Evans, G. W., Jamner, L. D., Davis, D. S., & Gärling, T. (2003). Tracking restoration in natural and urban field settings. Journal of Environmental Psychology, 23(2), 109-123.

[280] Kaplan, S. (1995). The restorative benefits of nature: Toward an integrative framework. Journal of Environmental Psychology, 15(3), 169-182.

Detoxification and Minimizing Environmental Toxins

Navigating Environmental Toxins: A Biohacker's Guide to Clean Living

Toxins in the environment can accumulate in your body and contribute to a range of health issues. We explore common sources of environmental toxins, from air and water pollutants to chemicals found in everyday products. Biohackers recognize the importance of minimizing toxin exposure to optimize their health.

Understanding Environmental Toxins

A. **Air Pollutants:**

- **Particulate Matter:** Fine particles in the air, often produced by combustion, can enter the lungs and bloodstream, contributing to respiratory and cardiovascular issues.[281]

- **Volatile Organic Compounds (VOCs):** Released by various products and materials, VOCs can lead to indoor air pollution and health problems.[282]

B. **Water Contaminants:**

- **Heavy Metals:** Lead, mercury, and arsenic can contaminate drinking water, posing serious health risks, particularly for children and pregnant women.[283]

[281] Brook, R. D., Rajagopalan, S., Pope, C. A., Brook, J. R., Bhatnagar, A., Diez-Roux, A. V., ... & Kaufman, J. D. (2010). Particulate matter air pollution and cardiovascular disease: An update to the scientific statement from the American Heart Association. Circulation, 121(21), 2331-2378.

[282] Mendell, M. J., Mirer, A. G., & Cheung, K. (2011). Respiratory and allergic health effects of dampness, mold, and dampness-related agents: A review of the epidemiologic evidence. Environmental Health Perspectives, 119(6), 748-756.

[283] Grandjean, P., & Landrigan, P. J. (2014). Neurobehavioural effects of developmental toxicity. The Lancet Neurology, 13(3), 330-338.

○ **Chemical Pollutants:** Pesticides, pharmaceuticals, and industrial chemicals may enter water sources, potentially impacting human health.[284]

C. Food Toxins:

○ **Pesticide Residues:** Consuming foods with pesticide residues can expose individuals to harmful chemicals, affecting the nervous system and hormone balance.[285]

○ **Food Additives:** Artificial preservatives, colorings, and flavor enhancers in processed foods may have adverse health effects.[286]

D. Everyday Products:

○ **Household Cleaners:** Many conventional cleaning products contain harsh chemicals that can irritate the skin, eyes, and respiratory system.[287]

○ **Personal Care Products:** Cosmetics and skincare products may contain toxic ingredients like phthalates, parabens, and synthetic fragrances.[288]

---

[284] Sirivarasai, J., Wananukul, W., Kaojarern, S., Chanprasertyothin, S., Thongmung, N., Ratanachaiwong, W., ... & Sura, T. (2012). Possible contamination of heavy metals in traditional Chinese medicines. Journal of Medical Toxicology, 8(4), 378-381.

[285] Chensheng, L. U., Colosio, C., & Fustinoni, S. (2014). Evidence of exposure to organophosphate pesticides in humans from urban and suburban areas: A review. Bulletin of Environmental Contamination and Toxicology, 93(5), 543-550.

[286] Schab, D. W., Trinh, N. H., Do, B. H., & Cau, D. Q. (2006). Artificial food colors in children in Vietnam: Prevalence, associated factors and behavioral effects. Food and Chemical Toxicology, 44(11), 1920-1923.

[287] Kim, J. L., Elfman, L., Mi, Y. W., Wieslander, G., Smedje, G., & Norbäck, D. (2007). Indoor molds, bacteria, microbial volatile organic compounds and plasticizers in schools—Associations with asthma and respiratory symptoms in pupils. Indoor Air, 17(2), 153-163.

[288] Darbre, P. D., Aljarrah, A., Miller, W. R., Coldham, N. G., Sauer, M. J., & Pope, G. S. (2004). Concentrations of parabens in human breast tumours. Journal of Applied Toxicology, 24(1), 5-13.

Biohackers and Toxin Minimization

A. **Dietary Choices:**

  o **Organic Foods:** Biohackers prioritize organic produce and avoid pesticide-laden options to reduce chemical exposure.[289]

  o **Filtered Water:** Using water filtration systems at home helps remove common contaminants from drinking water.[290]

B. **Non-Toxic Cleaning and Personal Care:**

  o **Natural Alternatives:** Biohackers opt for natural cleaning products and personal care items with transparent ingredient lists.[291]

  o **DIY Solutions:** Some biohackers create their cleaning and beauty products to have full control over ingredients.[292]

C. **Air Quality Enhancement:**

  o **Air Purification:** Using air purifiers at home can help reduce indoor air pollutants and improve air quality.[293]

  o **Ventilation:** Proper ventilation minimizes the accumulation of indoor pollutants.[294]

---

[289] Curl, C. L., Beresford, S. A., Fenske, R. A., Fitzpatrick, A. L., Lu, C., Nettleton, J. A., & Kaufman, J. D. (2015). Estimating pesticide exposure from dietary intake and organic food choices: The multi-ethnic study of atherosclerosis (MESA). Environmental Health Perspectives, 123(5), 475-483.

[290] Fawell, J., & Nieuwenhuijsen, M. J. Contaminants in drinking water: Environmental pollution and health. British Medical Bulletin, Volume 68, Issue 1, December 2003, pp. 199–208. https://doi.org/10.1093/bmb/ldg027

[291] Environmental Working Group. The dirty dozen: A look at toxic chemicals in household products. https://www.ewg.org/guides/cleaners/content/cleaners_and_health

[292] Campaign for Safe Cosmetics. Natural beauty: Evidence on ingredients and health effects. https://www.safecosmetics.org/get-the-facts/chemicals-of-concern/

[293] World Health Organization. Indoor air quality and health. https://www.who.int/news-room/fact-sheets/detail/indoor-air-pollution

[294] Environmental Protection Agency. Improving indoor air quality. https://www.epa.gov/indoor-air-quality-iaq

D. **Lifestyle Choices:**

  o **Reducing Plastic:** Biohackers limit plastic use and opt for glass or stainless-steel containers to avoid exposure to phthalates and BPA.[295]

  o **Detoxification Practices:** Some biohackers incorporate detox protocols, such as sauna sessions or intermittent fasting, to support toxin elimination.[296]

Advocating for Clean Living

A. **Regulatory Awareness:** Biohackers advocate for stricter regulations and transparency in the labeling of consumer products, urging governments and industries to prioritize health and safety.[297]

B. **Community Initiatives:** Engaging in local environmental projects and supporting clean living initiatives within communities fosters positive change.[298]

C. **Knowledge Sharing:** Biohackers contribute to collective knowledge by sharing research, experiences, and strategies to minimize toxin exposure for the benefit of all.[299]

Biohackers recognize that minimizing exposure to environmental toxins is not just a health choice; it's a way of life. By making informed decisions and taking proactive steps to reduce toxin exposure, they

---

[295] Center for International Environmental Law. Plastic and health: The hidden costs of a plastic planet. https://www.ciel.org/wp-content/uploads/2019/02/Plastic-and-Health-The-Hidden-Costs-of-a-Plastic-Planet-February-2019.pdf

[296] Eid, H. M., Nader, C., & Salem, D. E. Intermittent fasting: Is the wait worth the weight? https://www.ncbi.nlm.nih.gov/pmc/articles/PMC6128599/

[297] Safer Chemicals, Healthy Families. Chemicals of concern: Lobbying and advocacy. https://saferchemicals.org/learn/lobbying-and-advocacy/

[298] Marselle, M. R., Irvine, K. N., & Fuller, R. A. Community-based environmental initiatives: Challenges and opportunities. https://www.frontiersin.org/articles/10.3389/fenvs.2019.00023/full

[299]

strive to optimize their wellbeing and create a healthier environment for themselves and future generations.

Detoxification Strategies for Optimal Health

Practical strategies for detoxification include dietary choices, hydration, and specific detox protocols. Furthermore, the benefits of saunas, intermittent fasting, and liver support aid the body's natural detox processes. Biohackers understand that detoxification is an ongoing process that contributes to wellbeing.

Understanding Detoxification

1. **Liver Function:** The liver plays a central role in detoxification by metabolizing toxins and converting them into water-soluble compounds for excretion.[300]

2. **Elimination Pathways:** Toxins are eliminated through various pathways, including the liver, kidneys, skin, and digestive system.[301]

3. **Chronic Exposure:** Prolonged exposure to environmental toxins or poor dietary choices can overwhelm the body's natural detox mechanisms, leading to health issues.[302]

Practical Detoxification Strategies

1. **Hydration:**

   o **Importance of Water:** Staying well-hydrated is crucial for efficient toxin elimination through urine and sweat.[303]

[300] Kaplowitz, N. (2005). Mechanisms of liver cell injury. Journal of Hepatology, 42(1), 37–50.

[301] Pizzorno, J. ('014). Detoxification: A functional medicine approach. Integrative Medicine: A Clinician's Journal, 13(1), 8-10.

[302] Sears, M. E., Kerr, K. J., & Bray, R. I. (2012). Arsenic, cadmium, lead, and mercury in sweat: A systematic review. Journal of Environmental and Public Health, 2012.

[303] Popkin, B. M., D'Anci, K. E., & Rosenberg, I. H. (2010). Water, hydration, and health. Nutrition Reviews, 68(8), 439-458.

- **Lemon Water:** Drinking warm water with lemon in the morning can support liver function and digestion.[304]

- **Collagen/Hyaluronic Acid Matrix:** Drinking water is essential, but not enough. Replenishing hyaluronic acid in the body helps a lot with hydration.

2. Nutrient-Rich Diet:

- **Fruits and Vegetables:** A diet rich in plant-based foods provides essential vitamins, minerals, and antioxidants that support detoxification pathways.[305]

- **Fiber:** High-fiber foods promote regular bowel movements and help eliminate waste and toxins.[306]

3. Intermittent Fasting:

- **Fasting Benefits:** Intermittent fasting periods give the digestive system a rest and may enhance cellular autophagy, a process that removes damaged cells.[307]

- **Timing:** Various fasting protocols, such as the 16/8 method or periodic 24-hour fasts, can be adapted to individual preferences.[308]

---

[304] Kessler, H. S., Sisson, S. B., & Short, K. R. (2012). The potential for high-intensity interval training to reduce cardiometabolic disease risk. Sports Medicine, 42(6), 489-509.

[305] Liu, R. H. (2004). Potential synergy of phytochemicals in cancer prevention: Mechanism of action. Journal of Nutrition, 134(12), 3479S-3485S.

[306] Dahl, W. J., & Stewart, M. L. (2015). Position of the Academy of Nutrition and Dietetics: Health implications of dietary fiber. Journal of the Academy of Nutrition and Dietetics, 115(11), 1861-1870.

[307] Longo, V. D., & Mattson, M. P. (2014). Fasting: Molecular mechanisms and clinical applications. Cell Metabolism, 19(2), 181-192.

[308] Patterson, R. E., & Sears, D. D. (2017). Metabolic effects of intermittent fasting. Annual Review of Nutrition, 37, 371-393.

4. **Sauna Therapy:**
   - **Sweating Detox:** Sauna sessions induce sweating, which can help eliminate heavy metals and toxins through the skin.[309]
   - **Infrared Saunas:** Infrared heat penetrates deeper, promoting detoxification at the cellular level.[310]

5. **Liver Support:**
   - **Milk Thistle:** This herbal supplement may protect and support liver function, aiding detoxification.[311]
   - **Cruciferous Vegetables:** Foods like broccoli and Brussels sprouts contain compounds that boost liver detox enzymes.[312]

6. **Detox Protocols:**
   - **Juice Cleanses:** Short-term juice cleanses provide concentrated nutrients that support detoxification.[313]
   - **Detox Diets:** Structured detox diets focus on specific foods and may exclude potential allergens or inflammatory foods.[314]

---

[309] Crinnion, W. J. (2011). Sauna as a valuable clinical tool for cardiovascular, autoimmune, toxicant-induced and other chronic health problems. Alternative Medicine Review, 16(3), 215-225.

[310] Yu, S.Y., Chiu, J. H., Yang, S. D., Hsu, Y. C., Lui, W.Y., & Wu, C. W. (2006). Biological effect of far-infrared therapy on increasing skin microcirculation in rats. Photodermatology, Photoimmunology & Photomedicine, 22(2), 78-86.

[311] Abenavoli, L., Capasso, R., Milic, N., & Capasso, F. (2010). Milk thistle in liver diseases: Past, present, future. Phytotherapy Research, 24(10), 1423-1432.

[312] Pereira, C., Grácio, D., Teixeira, J. P., & Magro, F. (2017). Oxidative stress and DNA damage: Implications in inflammatory bowel disease. Inflammatory Bowel Diseases, 23(11), 1902-1917.

[313] Madsen, Lene et al. Juice fasting: An effective and safe approach for improving blood lipids. American Journal of Lifestyle Medicine. https://pubmed.ncbi.nlm.nih.gov/22407722/

[314] Klein, A.V., & Kiat, H. Detox diets for toxin elimination and weight management: A critical review of the evidence. Journal of Human Nutrition and Dietetics. https://pubmed.ncbi.nlm.nih.gov/25522674/

7. **Colon Hydrotherapy:**

- ○ **Colonic Irrigation:** This procedure involves flushing the colon with water to remove waste and toxins.[315]

- ○ **Professional Supervision:** Seek qualified practitioners for colon hydrotherapy sessions.

Biohackers and Personalized Detox

1. **Individualized Approach:** Biohackers tailor their detox strategies to their unique needs, goals, and sensitivities.[316]

2. **Monitoring and Testing:** Regular health assessments, such as liver function tests or toxin screenings, help biohackers track their progress.[317]

3. **Detox Mindset:** Embracing detoxification as an ongoing process rather than a one-time event supports long-term health optimization.[318]By incorporating these practical detoxification strategies into their lifestyle, biohackers aim to enhance their body's natural ability to remove toxins and promote good health.

---

[315] A. Ward, P. et al. Colon hydrotherapy: A review of the available evidence. Complementary Therapies in Clinical Practice. https://www.sciencedirect.com/science/article/abs/pii/S1744388112000905

B. Ernst, E. Safety of colonic irrigation: A systematic review and risk assessment. Journal of Alternative and Complementary Medicine. https://pubmed.ncbi.nlm.nih.gov/16722789/

[316] A. Ordovas, J. M., Ferguson, L. R., & Tai, E. S. et al. Personalized lifestyle medicine: Relevance for nutrition and lifestyle recommendations. Scientific Report of the 2016 ICAN Think Tank. https://www.ncbi.nlm.nih.gov/pmc/articles/PMC4933695/

B. Hayden, E. C. Personalized nutrition: Pioneering research offers promise for providing specific dietary advice based on individual genetic makeup. Nature. https://www.nature.com/articles/479039a

C. Harjutsalo, L. et al. The impact of personalized nutrition on chronic disease prevention and management: Outcomes from a scoping review. Nutrients. https://www.mdpi.com/2072-6643/12/8/2326

[317]

[318]

EMF Protection and Optimizing Your Home

Navigating EMF Exposure: Understanding its Impact on Health

The proliferation of electronic devices has led to increased exposure to electromagnetic fields (EMF), which may have adverse health effects. This section explores the science behind EMF exposure and its potential impact on sleep, cognition, and overall health. Biohackers take proactive steps to protect themselves from excessive EMF exposure.

The World of Electromagnetic Fields

1. **Sources of EMF:** EMFs originate from both natural (e.g., Earth's magnetic field) and human-made sources (e.g., cell phones, Wi-Fi, power lines).[319]

2. **Frequency Spectrum:** EMFs encompass a wide range of frequencies, from Extremely Low Frequency (ELF) to radiofrequency (RF) and microwave radiation.[320]

3. **Ionizing vs. Non-Ionizing:** EMFs are categorized as ionizing (high energy) or non-ionizing (low energy), with ionizing radiation carrying higher health risks.[321]

Potential Health Impacts of EMF Exposure

1. **Sleep Disruption:** EMF exposure, particularly from devices like smartphones and routers, has been linked to disrupted sleep patterns and reduced melatonin production.[322]

---

[319] Gandhi, O. P., & Kang, G. (2002). Some basic properties of electromagnetic fields. IEEE Engineering in Medicine and Biology Magazine, 21(6), 33–40.

[320] ICNIRP. (2020). ICNIRP guidelines for limiting exposure to electromagnetic fields. Health Physics, 118(5), 483–524.

[321] World Health Organization. (2018). What are electromagnetic fields? [Fact Sheet]. https://www.who.int/news-room/q-a-detail/radiation-electromagnetic-fields

[322] Higashikubo, R., Ragouzis, M., & Rappaport, S. M. (2001). Human sleep and EEG effects of 60-Hz magnetic fields. IEEE Engineering in Medicine and Biology Magazine, 20(3), 40–45.

2. **Cognitive Effects:** Some studies suggest that EMFs may impair cognitive functions, such as memory and attention, although the evidence is mixed.[323]

3. **Reproductive Health:** Emerging research explores the potential influence of EMFs on male fertility and female reproductive health.[324]

4. **Cancer Risk:** The association between EMF exposure and cancer, especially childhood leukemia, remains a subject of debate among scientists.[325]

Biohackers and EMF Mitigation

1. **EMF Awareness:** Biohackers prioritize understanding EMFs, their sources, and potential health effects through scientific research and expert guidance.[326]

2. **Safe Technology Use:**

   o **Distance:** Maintaining a safe distance from EMF-emitting devices reduces exposure.[327]

   o **Shielding:** EMF shielding products, such as Faraday cages or shielding fabrics, can block or reduce radiation.[328]

---

[323] Röösli, M., Frei, P., Mohler, E., & Hug, K. Systematic review on the health effects of exposure to radiofrequency electromagnetic fields from mobile phone base stations. (2010). Bulletin of the World Health Organization, 88(12), 887-896.

[324] Aitken, R. J., Bennetts, L. E., & Sawyer, D. (2005). Wiklendt, A., & King, B. V. Impact of radio frequency electromagnetic radiation on DNA integrity in the male germline. International Journal of Andrology, 28(3), 171-179.

[325] International Agency for Research on Cancer. (2013). IARC monographs on the evaluation of carcinogenic risks to humans. Volume 102: Non-Ionizing Radiation, Part 2: Radio-frequency Electromagnetic Fields.

[326] Biohacker's Handbook. (n.d.). Electromagnetic Fields. https://biohackingbook.com/chapters/emf/

[327] Sage, C., & Hardell, L. (2017). Increased brain cancer risk associated with wireless phone use. International Journal of Environmental Research and Public Health, 14(12), 1459.

[328] Lamech, F. (2019). Self-reporting of symptom development from exposure to radiofrequency fields of wireless smart meters in Victoria, Australia: A case series. Alternative Therapies in Health and Medicine, 25(1), 8-16.

3. **Sleep Hygiene:**
   - **Tech-Free Bedrooms:** Biohackers create EMF-free sleep environments by removing electronic devices or using shielded bedding.[329]

   - **EMF Meters:** Using EMF meters helps biohackers identify and mitigate high EMF areas in their homes.[330]

4. **Educational Advocacy:** Biohackers actively promote public awareness about the potential health impacts of EMFs and advocate for safer technologies.[331]

Future Research and Regulation

1. **Scientific Inquiry:** Ongoing research aims to clarify the health effects of EMF exposure, particularly concerning 5G technology and long-term exposure.[332]

2. **Regulatory Measures:** Biohackers may engage in efforts to advocate for stricter regulations on EMF-emitting devices and infrastructure.[333]

3. **Personalized Protection:** As individuals, biohackers explore and invest in EMF protection solutions tailored to their needs and concerns.[334]

---

[329] Zeichner, S. L. (2017). Is your bedroom EMF-free? How to reduce EMFs in the bedroom. Environmental Research, 159, 582-584.

[330] Trimmel, M., & Pachner, M. (2017). Electromagnetic field reduction restores health of electrosensitive people: An exploratory study. Electromagnetic Biology and Medicine, 36(3), 213-224.

[331] Environmental Health Trust. (n.d.). International actions on wireless. https://ehtrust.org/international-policy-actions-on-wireless/

[332] Miah, J., Sarran, C., & Gruzelier, J. (2017). Spatial working memory in mobile phone users. NeuroReport, 28(5), 239-243.

[333] Moskowitz, J. M. (2019). 5G wireless technology: Millimeter wave health effects. Environmental Research, 177, 108922.

[334] Havas, M. (2006). Electromagnetic hypersensitivity: Biological effects of dirty electricity with emphasis on diabetes and multiple sclerosis. Electromagnetic Biology and Medicine, 25(4), 259-268.

While the full extent of EMF's impact on human health continues to be studied, biohackers proactively employ strategies to reduce their EMF exposure, emphasizing the importance of sleep, cognition, and overall wellbeing in their journey toward optimal health.

Optimizing Your Home Environment for EMF Protection

We can optimize our home environment for EMF protection by minimizing wireless devices, using shielding materials, and creating EMF-free sleeping spaces. Biohackers prioritize the creation of a low-EMF home to support their wellbeing.

Understanding EMF Exposure at Home

1. **Sources of EMF:** Identify common sources of EMFs in your home, including Wi-Fi routers, cordless phones, smart meters, and electronic devices.[335]

2. **Wireless Technologies:** Recognize that wireless technologies such as Wi-Fi and Bluetooth emit radiofrequency (RF) radiation, contributing to EMF exposure.[336]

3. **Electrical Wiring:** Electrical wiring, especially in close proximity to living areas, can emit low-frequency EMFs known as extremely low-frequency (ELF) fields.[337]

---

[335] Electromagnetic Radiation Safety. (n.d.). How to reduce exposure to wireless radiation (EMF) sources. https://www.saferemr.com/2015/05/how-to-reduce-your-exposure-to-wireless.html

[336] Federal Communications Commission. (2015). Radiofrequency (RF) safety program. https://www.fcc.gov/general/radiofrequency-rf-safety-program

[337] BioInitiative Working Group. (2012). BioInitiative Report 2012: A rationale for biologically-based exposure standards for low-intensity electromagnetic radiation. https://bioinitiative.org/

Creating a Low-EMF Home

1. **Minimize Wireless Devices:**

   o **Ethernet Connections:** Use wired Ethernet connections instead of Wi-Fi whenever possible to reduce RF exposure.[338]

   o **Airplane Mode:** Switch devices to airplane mode at night to reduce RF radiation.

2. **Shielding Materials:**

   o **EMF Paint:** Consider painting walls with EMF shielding paint, which blocks RF radiation.[339]

   o **Window Films:** Apply window films containing metal or carbon to reduce incoming RF radiation.[340]

3. **Bedroom EMF Sanctuary:**

   o **Turn off Wi-Fi:** Disable Wi-Fi routers at night or place them in a room far from the bedroom.[341]

   o **EMF-Free Bedding:** Invest in EMF-blocking bedding, including canopy nets and blankets.[342]

4. **Reduce Dirty Electricity:**

   o **Filter Installation:** Install dirty electricity filters to minimize high-frequency transients on electrical lines.[343]

---

[338] Havas, M., & Marrongelle, J. (2013). Reducing wireless radiation exposure in schools: A parent guide. Environmental Health Trust. https://ehtrust.org/wp-content/uploads/2015/11/Reducing-Wireless-Radiation-Exposure-in-Schools-Overview.pdf

[339] Ecomad. (n.d.). EMF shielding paint: Protect your home from EMF radiation. https://ecomad.biz/products/emf-shielding-paint

[340] LessEMF. (n.d.). Window films. https://www.lessemf.com/window.html

[341] Safe Living Technologies. (n.d.). EMF meter, dirty electricity, and electrosmog detectors. https://slt.co/Products/Room-EMF-Detectors

[342] EMF Protection Store. (n.d.). EMF shielding canopy bed curtain. https://www.emfprotectionstore.com/emfshieldingbed.html

[343] Stetzer Electric. (n.d.). Stetzer filters. https://www.stetzerelectric.com/stetzerfilters/

○ **Limit Devices:** Reduce the number of plugged-in electronic devices and use battery-operated alternatives when possible.

5. **Smart Meter Safety:**

○ **Opt-Out Options:** Inquire about smart meter opt-out programs or consider shielding solutions.[344]

○ **Distance:** Maintain a safe distance from smart meters, especially in bedrooms or frequently used spaces.

Biohackers and EMF Mitigation

1. **Educational Advocacy:** Biohackers share knowledge about EMF protection strategies and advocate for responsible technology use within their communities.[345]

2. **Measurement Tools:** Utilize EMF meters to assess and monitor EMF levels in your home, identifying areas of concern for mitigation.[346]

3. **Personalized Solutions:** Tailor EMF protection measures to your specific needs, taking into account individual sensitivities and concerns.[347]

By adopting these techniques and creating a low-EMF home environment, biohackers strive to reduce their EMF exposure and support their overall wellbeing, emphasizing the importance of quality sleep, cognitive function, and long-term health.

---

[344] Smart Grid Awareness. (n.d.). What is a smart meter? https://smartgridawareness.org/about/smart-meters/what-is-a-smart-meter/

[345] Electromagnetic Radiation Safety. (n.d.). Advocacy. https://www.saferemr.com/p/advocacy.html

[346] Malegiannakis, I. E., Lampropoulou, A. M., & Karipidis, T. A. et al. Measurement techniques and mitigation strategies for electromagnetic field exposures in indoor environments. Energies. https://www.mdpi.com/1996-1073/14/2/365

[347]

Sustainable Living: Biohackers and Environmental Consciousness

The Interconnectedness of Personal and Planetary Health

Sustainability is a critical aspect of biohacking for the future. We explore the importance of reducing environmental impact through eco-friendly practices such as minimalism, renewable energy adoption, and waste reduction. Biohackers recognize the interconnectedness of personal and planetary health.

1. **Holistic Perspective:** Biohackers embrace a holistic perspective that recognizes the interdependence of personal health, community wellbeing, and environmental sustainability.[348]

2. **Global Impact:** They acknowledge that individual choices can have a significant impact on global environmental issues such as climate change, resource depletion, and pollution.[349]

Practices for Sustainable Living

1. **Minimalism:**

   o **Conscious Consumption:** Biohackers prioritize mindful and intentional consumption, focusing on quality over quantity.[350]

---

[348] Seltenrich, N. (2015). Just one thing: Environmental determinants of human health. Environmental Health Perspectives, 123(12), A296–A303.

[349] IPCC. (2014). Climate Change 2014: Synthesis Report. Contribution of Working Groups I, II and III to the Fifth Assessment Report of the Intergovernmental Panel on Climate Change. https://www.ipcc.ch/site/assets/uploads/2018/02/SYR_AR5_FINAL_full_wcover.pdf

[350] Sartore, M. L., & Cunningham, T. R. (2019). Consuming sustainability: A review of the role of mindfulness as a personal virtue and consumer good. Sustainable Production and Consumption, 19, 149-158.

○ **Decluttering:** Minimalism extends to decluttering physical and mental spaces, promoting mental clarity and reducing stress.[351]

2. **Renewable Energy Adoption:**

   ○ **Solar Power:** Installing solar panels at home reduces reliance on fossil fuels and lowers carbon emissions.[352]

   ○ **Wind Energy:** Exploring wind energy options contributes to a sustainable energy mix.[353]

3. **Waste Reduction:**

   ○ **Zero-Waste Living:** Biohackers embrace the zero-waste lifestyle, reducing, reusing, and recycling to minimize waste.[354]

   ○ **Composting:** Composting organic waste reduces landfill contributions and enriches soil.[355]

4. **Plant-Based Diets:**

   ○ **Environmental Impact:** Transitioning to plant-based diets reduces greenhouse gas emissions, land use, and water consumption.[356]

---

[351] Anderson, C. (2016). The impact of minimalism on consumers' emotional wellbeing. The Journal of Consumer Affairs, 50(1), 121-147.

[352] Jacobson, M. Z. (2009). Review of solutions to global warming, air pollution, and energy security. Energy and Environmental Science, 2(2), 148-173.

[353] Archer, C. L., & Jacobson, M. Z. (2005). Evaluation of global wind power. Journal of Geophysical Research: Atmospheres, 110(D12).

[354] Nørgaard, K., & Laugesen, J. S. (2019). Zero waste and the politics of a circular economy: Some critical perspectives. Environmental Innovation and Societal Transitions, 33, 49-55.

[355] Bernal-Brooks, F. W., & Broadhead, A. (2017). Compost benefits for agriculture and the environment. In Soil Amendments (pp. 33-62). IntechOpen.

[356] Springmann, M., Godfray, H. C. J., Rayner, M., & Scarborough, P. (2016). Analysis and valuation of the health and climate change cobenefits of dietary change. Proceedings of the National Academy of Sciences, 113(15), 4146-4151.

○ **Personal Health:** Plant-based diets are associated with numerous health benefits, aligning with biohackers' focus on wellbeing.[357]

5. **Active Transportation:**

○ **Biking and Walking:** Opting for active transportation modes reduces carbon emissions and promotes physical activity.[358]

○ **Public Transit:** Using public transportation contributes to lower vehicle emissions and decreased traffic congestion.[359]

Biohackers as Eco-Citizens

1. **Environmental Advocacy:** Biohackers often engage in advocacy efforts, supporting policies and initiatives aimed at sustainability and conservation.[360]

2. **Community Building:** They encourage eco-conscious communities that share sustainable living practices and create a supportive environment.[361]

3. **Education and Awareness:** Biohackers actively educate themselves and others about the environmental impact of personal choices, driving positive change.[362]

---

[357] Dinu, M., Abbate, R., Gensini, G. F., Casini, A., & Sofi, F. (2017). Vegetarian, vegan diets and multiple health outcomes: A systematic review with meta-analysis of observational studies. Critical Reviews in Food Science and Nutrition, 57(17), 3640-3649.

[358] Gössling, S., Scott, D., & Hall, C. M. (2020). Tourism and water: Interactions and impacts. Channel View Publications.

[359] Litman, T. (2019). Transportation and Public Health. Victoria Transport Policy Institute.

[360] Honeck, R. P., Nöllenburg, M., Rutter, I., & Wolff, A. (2017). A new heuristic for the Chinese postman problem with multiple routes. Computers & Operations Research, 78, 262-277.

[361] Frumkin, H. (2017). Environmental health: From global to local. John Wiley & Sons.

[362] Hossain, M. N., & Faizal, H. M. (2020). Green consumption and environmental awareness: Willingness to pay for eco-friendly products in Bangladesh. Journal of Cleaner Production, 268, 121831.

By integrating eco-friendly practices into their lifestyles, biohackers not only optimize their personal wellbeing but also contribute to a healthier, more sustainable planet. They recognize that the pursuit of optimal health extends beyond the individual to encompass the global ecosystem.

Sustainable Food Choices: Aligning Biohacking with Eco-Conscious Practices

Biohackers are committed to leaving a positive impact on the planet, including sustainable food choices, ethical sourcing, and eco-conscious practices that align with biohacking principles. By making choices that benefit both individual health and the environment, biohackers contribute to a sustainable future.

The Intersection of Health and Sustainability

1. **Nutrient-Dense Foods:** Biohackers prioritize nutrient-dense whole foods, emphasizing the importance of organic fruits and vegetables, whole grains, and lean proteins.[363]

2. **Local and Seasonal Produce:** They choose locally sourced and seasonal foods to reduce the carbon footprint associated with transportation and support local agriculture.[364]

3. **Plant-Based Diets:** Many biohackers embrace plant-based diets, not only for their health benefits but also for the reduced environmental impact associated with lower meat consumption.[365]

---

[363] Drewnowski, A., & Almiron-Roig, E. (2010). Human perceptions and preferences for fat and sugar in foods. In Montmayeur J.P., le Coutre J., & Sclafani A. (Eds.). Fat detection: Taste, texture, and post ingestive effects (pp. 265-290). CRC Press/Taylor & Francis.

[364] Macdiarmid, J. I., Kyle, J., & Horgan, G. W. (2012). Sustainable diets for the future: Can we contribute to reducing greenhouse gas emissions by eating a healthy diet? The American Journal of Clinical Nutrition, 96(3), 632-639.

[365] Sabaté, J., Soret, S., & Sustainability of Plant-Based Diets: Back to the future. (2014). The American Journal of Clinical Nutrition, 100(Supplement_1), 476S-482S.

Ethical Sourcing and Eco-Conscious Practices

1. **Sustainable Farming Practices:**

   o **Organic Farming:** Biohackers support organic farming methods that prioritize soil health, biodiversity, and reduced chemical use.[366]

   o **Regenerative Agriculture:** They advocate for regenerative farming practices that restore soil health, sequester carbon, and enhance ecosystem resilience.[367]

2. **Ethical Animal Farming:**

   o **Pasture-Raised:** When choosing animal products, biohackers opt for pasture-raised and humanely raised options.[368]

   o **Wild-Caught Seafood:** They prioritize sustainably harvested seafood to protect marine ecosystems.[369]

3. **Minimizing Food Waste:**

   o **Meal Planning:** Biohackers plan meals to reduce food waste and make the most of ingredients.[370]

   o **Composting:** They compost food scraps to divert organic waste from landfills and enrich soil.[371]

---

[366] Reganold, J. P., Wachter, J. M., & Organic agriculture in the twenty-first century. (2016). Nature Plants, 2(2), 15221.

[367] Lal, R. (2015). Restoring soil quality to mitigate soil degradation. Sustainability, 7(5), 5875-5895.

[368] Rodale Institute. (n.d.). Pasture-raised standards. https://rodaleinstitute.org/regenerative-organic-practices/pasture-raised-standards/

[369] Monterey Bay Aquarium Seafood Watch. (2021). Our science. https://www.seafood-watch.org/seafood-recommendations/our-science

[370] Gustavsson, J., Cederberg, C., Sonesson, U., van Otterdijk, R., & Meybeck, A. (2011). Global food losses and food waste: Extent, causes, and prevention. FAO.

[371] Environmental Protection Agency. (2021). Sustainable management of food. https://www.epa.gov/sustainable-management-food/sustainable-management-food-basics

Biohackers and Sustainable Eating Habits

1. **Personalized Nutrition:** Biohackers tailor their diets to their unique needs, experimenting with various approaches to find what works best for them.[372]

2. **Educational Advocacy:** They actively educate themselves and others about the environmental impact of dietary choices and advocate for sustainable practices.[373]

3. **Local Community Engagement:** Biohackers often engage with local food initiatives, such as community-supported agriculture (CSA) programs and farmers' markets.[374]

By aligning their dietary choices with eco-conscious practices, biohackers promote a sustainable food system that benefits both individual health and the health of the planet. They recognize that the pursuit of optimal health extends beyond personal wellbeing to include responsible stewardship of the environment.

Biohacking your environment is a holistic approach to optimizing health and wellbeing. By understanding these key factors, you can create an environment that nurtures your health and contributes to a thriving, eco-conscious world.

---

[372] Shuval, K., & Brzoska, P. (2017). Dietary recommendations for health and the environment: A conflict of interest? Critical Public Health, 27(5), 599-609.

[373] Borgstrom, E., & Cederberg, C. (2020). Climate-smart diets for a sustainable planet: A systematic review. Advances in Nutrition, 11(4), 828-846.

[374] Willett, W., Rockström, J., Loken, B., Springmann, M., Lang, T., Vermeulen, S., ... & Murray, C. J. L. (2019). Food in the Anthropocene: The EAT–Lancet Commission on healthy diets from sustainable food systems. The Lancet, 393(10170), 447-492.

CHAPTER 9

BIOHACKING FOR MENTAL HEALTH

In a world marked by the fast pace of modern life, mental health has become a crucial focus for biohackers. This chapter explores various biohacking techniques and strategies to enhance mental well-being. From stress management techniques to the fascinating world of biofeedback, psychedelics, and the vital role of community and connection, biohackers employ multifaceted approaches to optimize mental health.

Stress Management Techniques

The Vicious Cycle: Chronic Stress and Mental Health

Stress is a ubiquitous and often detrimental force in our lives. We must examine the pervasive impact of stress on mental health, exploring how chronic stress contributes to anxiety, depression, and other mental health issues.

Unraveling the Stress-Mental Health Connection

Stress, in its essence, is a natural response that prepares our bodies to tackle challenges. It prompts the release of hormones like cortisol and adrenaline, gearing us up for action.[375] While acute stress can be adaptive and even beneficial, chronic stress, characterized by the persistent activation of the body's stress response, can have profound and detrimental effects.[376]

Chronic Stress's Impact on Mental Health

1. **Anxiety Disorders:** One of the most striking connections is the link between chronic stress and anxiety disorders. It significantly increases the risk of conditions like generalized anxiety disorder (GAD) and panic disorder, making daily life a constant struggle.[377]

2. **Depression:** Prolonged stress can lead to alterations in brain chemistry, rendering individuals more susceptible to depression. It's as if chronic stress chips away at the brain's resilience.[378]

3. **Post-Traumatic Stress Disorder (PTSD):** Chronic stress, particularly in the form of traumatic experiences, can set the stage for the development of PTSD, a condition that profoundly affects an individual's mental wellbeing.[379]

The Neurobiological Underpinnings

1. **Hippocampus and Amygdala:** Chronic stress can bring about structural changes in the brain, particularly in regions

---

[375] McEwen, B. S., & Sapolsky, R. M. (1995). Stress and cognitive function. Current Opinion in Neurobiology, 5(2), 205-216.

[376] Lupien, S. J., McEwen, B. S., Gunnar, M. R., & Heim, C. (2009). Effects of stress throughout the lifespan on the brain, behaviour and cognition. Nature Reviews Neuroscience, 10(6), 434-445.

[377] McLaughlin, K. A., & Nolen-Hoeksema, S. (2011). Rumination as a transdiagnostic factor in depression and anxiety. Behaviour Research and Therapy, 49(3), 186-193.

[378] Hovatta, I., Tennant, R. S., Helton, R., Marr, R. A., Singer, O., Redwine, J. M., ... & Weissman, I. L. (2005). Glyoxalase 1 and glutathione reductase 1 regulate anxiety in mice. Nature, 438(7068), 662-666.

[379] Yehuda, R., & LeDoux, J. (2007). Response variation following trauma: A translational neuroscience approach to understanding PTSD. Neuron, 56(1), 19-32.

such as the hippocampus and amygdala. These areas play pivotal roles in regulating mood, and stress-induced alterations can have profound implications.[380]

2. **Neurotransmitter Imbalance:** Stress disrupts the delicate balance of neurotransmitters like serotonin and dopamine, contributing to the onset of mood disorders like anxiety and depression.[381]

The Stress-Health Connection: Biohacker Strategies

Biohackers are acutely aware of the significance of stress management in optimizing their overall wellbeing. They employ a range of techniques to keep chronic stress at bay:

A. **Stress Management Techniques:** Biohackers prioritize practices like mindfulness meditation, deep breathing exercises, and progressive muscle relaxation to keep stress levels in check.[382]

B. **Physical Activity:** Regular exercise is a cornerstone of biohacking. It helps to reduce stress hormones and triggers the release of endorphins, the body's natural mood lifters.[383]

C. **Sleep Optimization:** Adequate, high-quality sleep is crucial for stress resilience and maintaining good mental health. Biohackers employ strategies to enhance their sleep, ensuring they wake up refreshed and ready to face the day.[384]

---

[380] Sapolsky, R. M. (1996). Why stress is bad for your brain. Science, 273(5276), 749-750.

[381] Pariante, C. M., & Lightman, S. L. (2008). The HPA axis in major depression: Classical theories and new developments. Trends in Neurosciences, 31(9), 464-468.

[382] Hofmann, S. G., Asnaani, A., Vonk, I. J., Sawyer, A. T., & Fang, A. (2012). The efficacy of cognitive behavioral therapy: A review of meta-analyses. Cognitive Therapy and Research, 36(5), 427-440.

[383] Salmon, P. (2001). Effects of physical exercise on anxiety, depression, and sensitivity to stress: A unifying theory. Clinical Psychology Review, 21(1), 33-61.

[384] Walker, M. P. (2017). Why We Sleep: The New Science of Sleep And Dreams. Penguin.

D. **Nutrition:** Nutrient-dense diets, rich in antioxidants and anti-inflammatory foods, support the brain's resilience to stress. What you eat can significantly impact how you feel.[385]

E. **Supplementation:** Biohackers may explore the use of adaptogenic herbs, omega-3 fatty acids, and other supplements that support the body's ability to adapt to stress.[386]

Seeking Professional Help

Biohackers understand the value of seeking professional help when needed:

A. **Therapy:** Many biohackers recognize the efficacy of therapy, including cognitive-behavioral therapy (CBT) and other evidence-based approaches, in managing stress and mental health. Talking to a trained therapist can provide valuable insights and strategies for coping with stress.[387]

B. **Medication:** In some cases, medication prescribed by healthcare professionals may be necessary to manage severe stress-related disorders. Biohackers prioritize their mental health and are open to discussing medication options when appropriate.[388]

---

[385] Jacka, F. N., Mykletun, A., Berk, M., Bjelland, I., & Tell, G. S. (2011). The association between habitual diet quality and the common mental disorders in community-dwelling adults: The Hordaland Health study. Psychosomatic Medicine, 73(6), 483-490.

[386] Panossian, A., & Wikman, G. (2010). Effects of adaptogens on the central nervous system and the molecular mechanisms associated with their stress-protective activity. Pharmaceuticals, 3(1), 188-224.

[387] Butler, A. C., Chapman, J. E., Forman, E. M., & Beck, A. T. (2006). The empirical status of cognitive-behavioral therapy: A review of meta-analyses. Clinical Psychology Review, 26(1), 17-31.

[388] Rush, AI., Trivedi, M. H., Wisniewski, S. R., Nierenberg, A. A., Stewart, J. W., Warden, D., ... & Fava, M. (2006). Acute and longer-term outcomes in depressed outpatients requiring one or several treatment steps: A STAR*D report. The American Journal of Psychiatry, 163(11), 1905-1917.

By comprehending the profound impact of chronic stress on mental health and employing biohacking strategies to mitigate its effects, biohackers strive to optimize their mental wellbeing and overall health.

Stress Management Techniques: Building Mental Resilience

Biohackers recognize that managing stress is essential for mental wellbeing. Practical stress management techniques include mindfulness meditation, deep breathing exercises, and progressive muscle relaxation. These techniques empower us to regain control over our stress response and promote mental resilience.

Mindfulness Meditation: The Art of Present Awareness

Mindfulness meditation is a practice that invites individuals to immerse themselves fully in the present moment, observing their thoughts and emotions without judgment. It's a gentle voyage into self-awareness and tranquility.[389]

- **Stress Reduction:** Mindfulness meditation offers profound stress reduction benefits by promoting relaxation and bolstering emotional regulation. It helps individuals find their center amidst life's turbulence.[390]

- **Practical Guidance:** The fundamentals of mindfulness meditation include establishing the right posture and mastering mindful breathing techniques.[391]

---

[389] Kabat-Zinn, J. (1994). Wherever You Go, There You Are: Mindfulness Meditation in Everyday Life. Hachette Books.

[390] Hofmann, S. G., Sawyer, A. T., Witt, A. A., & Oh, D. (2010). The effect of mindfulness-based therapy on anxiety and depression: A meta-analytic review. Journal of Consulting and Clinical Psychology, 78(2), 169–183.

[391] Harris, R. (2009). ACT Made Simple: An Easy-To-Read Primer on Acceptance and Commitment Therapy. New Harbinger Publications.

Posture:

- **Sit or Lie Down:** Find a comfortable and stable position. You can sit cross-legged on a cushion, a chair, or even lie down, depending on what feels most comfortable.

- **Straighten Your Spine:** Maintain an upright but relaxed posture. This allows for easy breathing and alertness.

- **Hands and Legs:** Rest your hands on your lap or knees. If sitting, you can place your hands palms down or palms up. Keep your legs in a comfortable position, either crossed or with your feet flat on the floor.

- **Eyes:** Close your eyes gently or keep them partially open with a soft gaze on a point in front of you. Experiment with what works best for you.

Mindful Breathing Techniques:

- **Focus on Your Breath:** Pay attention to your breath as it naturally flows in and out of your nostrils or the rise and fall of your abdomen or chest.

- **Observe without Judgment:** If your mind wanders, gently bring your focus back to your breath without criticizing yourself. Mindfulness is about non-judgmental awareness. **Counting breaths:** Some people find it helpful to count breaths, such as silently counting "one" on the inhale and "two" on the exhale, up to a certain number (e.g., five) and then starting over.

- **Body Scan:** Instead of focusing solely on the breath, you can also practice a body scan. Start from the top of your head and gradually move your attention down through your body, noticing any sensations or tension.

Integrating Mindfulness into Everyday Life:

- **Mindful Eating:** Pay full attention to the taste, texture, and smell of your food during meals. Avoid distractions like phones or TV.

- **Mindful Walking:** When walking, be present in each step, feeling the ground beneath your feet and the movement of your body. It can turn a routine activity into a mindfulness exercise.

- **Mindful Breaks:** Take short mindfulness breaks throughout the day. Pause for a minute or two to focus on your breath and bring your attention back to the present moment.

- **Mindful Listening:** When in conversations, truly listen to the person speaking without thinking about your response. This can enhance your communication and connection with others.

- **Mindful Routines:** Incorporate mindfulness into daily routines like brushing your teeth, showering, or waiting in line by being fully present during these activities.

- **Mindful Reminders:** Set reminders on your phone or use objects in your environment to trigger moments of mindfulness. When you see or hear these reminders, briefly pause to center yourself.

  Remember that mindfulness is a skill that requires practice. Start with short sessions and gradually extend the duration as you become more comfortable. Consistency is key to experiencing the benefits of mindfulness meditation, and integrating mindfulness into your daily life can help you maintain a more present and peaceful state of mind.

Deep Breathing Exercises: The Breath of Serenity

Deep breathing exercises are wonderfully simple yet potent tools for managing stress. They operate by activating the body's relaxation response through focused and intentional breathing techniques.[392]

- **The Art of Breath:** Various deep breathing methods include diaphragmatic breathing and the renowned 4-7-8 technique.[393]
- **Incorporating Deep Breathing:** Practicality is key. You can effortlessly weave deep breathing exercises into your daily routines, whether it's for a quick moment of calm at work or a tranquil pre-sleep relaxation ritual.[394]

Progressive Muscle Relaxation: Easing Tensions, Body, and Mind

Chronic stress often manifests as muscle tension, a physical representation of our inner turmoil. Progressive muscle relaxation is a structured approach to relieving this tension, involving the systematic tensing and releasing of muscle groups to promote physical and mental relaxation.[395]

- **Step-by-Step Practice:** A progressive muscle relaxation session helps to deepen the understanding of the process and its therapeutic benefits.[396]
- **Incorporating Regular Practice:** Progressive muscle relaxation should be a regular part of your daily routine. By doing so, you can reduce stress-related muscle tension and enhance relaxation.[397]

---

[392] Jerath, R., Edry, J. W., Barnes, V. A., & Jerath, V. (2006). Physiology of long pranayamic breathing: Neural respiratory elements may provide a mechanism that explains how slow deep breathing shifts the autonomic nervous system. Medical Hypotheses, 67(3), 566–571.

[393] McCall, T. (2012). Yoga as Medicine: The Yogic Prescription for Health and Healing. Bantam.

[394] Ross, A., & Thomas, S. (2010). The health benefits of yoga and exercise: A review of comparison studies. The Journal of Alternative and Complementary Medicine, 16(1), 3–12.

[395] Bernstein, D. A., & Borkovec, T. D. (1973). Progressive Relaxation Training: A Manual for the Helping Professions. Research Press.

[396] Jacobson, E. (1938). Progressive Relaxation: A Physiological and Clinical Investigation of Muscular States and Their Significance in Psychology and Medical Practice. University of Chicago Press.

[397] Bernstein, D. A., & Borkovec, T. D. (1973). Progressive Relaxation Training: A Manual for the Helping Professions. Research Press.

Biohacker Strategies: Elevating Stress Management Techniques

Biohackers wholeheartedly recognize the value of these stress management techniques. Furthermore, they employ these practices as indispensable tools in their daily routines to enhance mental resilience and maintain peak performance.[398]

Integration of Technology: Technology can augment the effectiveness of these techniques. Biohackers often utilize meditation apps and heart rate variability (HRV) monitoring to fine-tune their stress management approaches.[399]

By embracing mindfulness meditation, deep breathing exercises, and progressive muscle relaxation, you can empower yourself to reclaim control over your stress responses. These practices not only offer immediate relief from the rigors of daily life but also contribute to long-term mental resilience, enabling you to thrive even in the face of life's most formidable challenges.

Biofeedback and Neurofeedback

Biohacker's Guide to Optimizing Vital Signs and Mental Health

Biofeedback and neurofeedback are cutting-edge tools that provide real-time information about physiological processes, helping individuals gain control over their mental and emotional states. We explore how biohackers use these techniques to regulate heart rate, brainwave patterns, and other vital signs, ultimately enhancing their mental health.

---

[398] Asprey, D. (2019). Game Changers: What Leaders, Innovators, and Mavericks Do to Win at Life. Harper Wave.

[399] Chittaro, L., & Sioni, R. (2014). Evaluation of a mobile mindfulness app distributed through on-line stores: A 4-week study. International Journal of Human-Computer Interaction, 30(2), 89-102.

Mindful Mastery of Vital Signs

Biohackers understand that the mind and body are intricately linked. Through mindfulness meditation, they gain the ability to influence vital signs consciously:

- **Heart Rate Mastery:** Mindfulness meditation, with its focus on breath and awareness, empowers biohackers to regulate their heart rate. They can navigate from a state of heightened stress to one of calm and equilibrium with ease.[400]

- **Blood Pressure Balance:** As their mindfulness practice deepens, biohackers often notice a remarkable reduction in their blood pressure levels. This promotes cardiovascular health and fosters a sense of tranquility and wellbeing.[401]

Brainwave Harmony and Mental Resilience

Biohackers recognize that mental resilience is closely tied to brainwave patterns. They employ stress management techniques to achieve synchronization:

- **Brainwave Synchronization:** Deep breathing exercises and mindfulness meditation are powerful tools for synchronizing brainwave patterns. They help biohackers transition from active beta states to the more relaxed and creative alpha and theta states, enhancing mental clarity and emotional resilience.[402]

---

[400] Tang, Y. Y., Ma, Y., Fan, Y., Feng, H., Wang, J., Feng, S., ... & Posner, M. I. (2009). Central and autonomic nervous system interaction is altered by short-term meditation. Proceedings of the National Academy of Sciences, 106(22), 8865-8870.

[401] Anderson, J. W., Liu, C., & Kryscio, R. J. (2008). Blood pressure response to transcendental meditation: A meta-analysis. American Journal of Hypertension, 21(3), 310-316.

[402] Travis, F., & Shear, J. (2010). Focused attention, open monitoring and automatic self-transcending: Categories to organize meditations from Vedic, Buddhist and Chinese traditions. Consciousness and Cognition, 19(4), 1110-1118.

- **Cortical Coherence:** Progressive muscle relaxation, a favored technique, enhances cortical coherence. This synchronization between different brain regions contributes to better decision-making, emotional stability, and overall cognitive function.[403]

Elevating Mental Health

Biohackers prioritize their mental health and leverage these techniques for substantial gains:

- **Stress Reduction:** By consistently practicing mindfulness meditation and related techniques, biohackers report significant reductions in stress-related symptoms. Anxiety, depression, and psychological distress are notably diminished.[404]

- **Enhanced Emotional Regulation:** With mindfulness as their ally, biohackers develop heightened emotional intelligence and regulation. They are better equipped to navigate complex emotions, maintaining equilibrium even in turbulent times.[405]

Quantifying Mental Health Progress

Biohackers are data-driven, and they use technology to quantify their mental health improvements:

- **Heart Rate Variability (HRV):** HRV becomes a quantitative marker of mental health and stress resilience. Biohackers

---

[403] Cannon, R. L., & Lubar, J. F. (2007). EEG spectral power and coherence: Differentiating effects of spatial–temporal tasks in children with and without ADHD. Clinical Neurophysiology, 118(10), 2225-2241.

[404] Hofmann, S. G., Sawyer, A. T., Witt, A. A., & Oh, D. (2010). The effect of mindfulness-based therapy on anxiety and depression: A meta-analytic review. Journal of Consulting and Clinical Psychology, 78(2), 169-183.

[405] Goldin, P. R., & Gross, J. J. (2010). Effects of mindfulness-based stress reduction (MBSR) on emotion regulation in social anxiety disorder. Emotion, 10(1), 83-91.

employ biofeedback devices to monitor and optimize their HRV, gaining insights into their overall wellbeing.[406]

- **Neurofeedback:** Some biohackers delve into neurofeedback technologies, allowing them to directly train their brainwave patterns for improved mental health outcomes. This data-centric approach aligns perfectly with their biohacking philosophy.[407]

Thriving Through Biohacked Mental Resilience

By embracing mindfulness meditation, deep breathing exercises, and progressive muscle relaxation, biohackers embark on a transformative journey toward self-mastery and mental resilience. They skillfully regulate vital signs, harmonize brainwave patterns, and fortify their emotional wellbeing. Through continuous practice and the judicious use of technology, biohackers aim not only to unlock their mental potential but also to thrive in the face of life's challenges.

Biofeedback and Neurofeedback: Pioneering Mental Wellbeing

Biohackers understand that data is key to optimization. Biofeedback and neurofeedback empower individuals to track their mental and emotional states, making it possible to identify patterns and develop personalized strategies for mental wellbeing.

Biofeedback: A Window into the Mind and Body

Biofeedback is a groundbreaking technology that provides real-time data on physiological processes, allowing individuals to gain insights into their mental and emotional states:

[406] Lehrer, P. M., & Gevirtz, R. (2014). Heart rate variability biofeedback: How and why does it work? Frontiers in Psychology, 5, 756.

[407] Vernon, D. (2005). Can neurofeedback training enhance performance? An evaluation of the evidence with implications for future research. Applied Psychophysiology and Biofeedback, 30(4), 347-364.

1. **Understanding Physiology:** Biofeedback devices measure parameters like heart rate, skin conductivity, and muscle tension. By receiving immediate feedback on these variables, individuals gain a deeper understanding of how their bodies respond to stress and emotions.[408]

2. **Identifying Stress Patterns:** Through regular biofeedback sessions, biohackers can identify patterns in their physiological responses to stressors. This data-driven approach helps them recognize triggers and develop tailored stress management techniques.[409]

3. **Personalized Stress Management:** Armed with the knowledge acquired through biofeedback, individuals can fine-tune their stress management strategies. They may incorporate mindfulness meditation, deep breathing exercises, or progressive muscle relaxation based on their unique physiological responses.[410]

Neurofeedback: Rewiring the Brain for Mental Resilience

Neurofeedback takes the concept further by directly training the brain's electrical activity. It allows individuals to:

1. **Brainwave Regulation:** Neurofeedback systems measure brainwave patterns and provide real-time feedback. Biohackers can learn to regulate these patterns, shifting from states of stress and anxiety to those of relaxation and focus.[411]

---

[408] Yucha, C., & Montgomery, D. (2008). Evidence-Based Practice in Biofeedback and Neurofeedback. AAPB.

[409] Moss, D., McGrady, A., Davies, T. C., & Wickramasekera, I. E. (2005). The Handbook of Mind-Body Medicine for Primary Care: A Holistic Approach to Efficacy. Sage.

[410] Khazan, I. Z. (2013). The Clinical Handbook of Biofeedback: A Step-by-Step Guide for Training and Practice with Mindfulness. Wiley.

[411] Hammond, D. C. (2010). Neurofeedback with anxiety and affective disorders. Child and Adolescent Psychiatric Clinics, 19(2), 245-265

2. **Enhancing Emotional Resilience:** Neurofeedback sessions enable individuals to rewire their brains for enhanced emotional resilience. By strengthening areas associated with emotional regulation, they can better manage stress and negative emotions.[412]

3. **Optimizing Cognitive Function:** Biohackers often use neurofeedback to optimize cognitive function. By enhancing brainwave patterns associated with memory, creativity, and problem-solving, they can boost mental performance.[413]

Personalized Mental Wellbeing Strategies

The true power of biofeedback and neurofeedback lies in personalization:

1. **Data-Driven Insights:** These technologies provide data-driven insights into an individual's mental and emotional states. By tracking changes over time, patterns and trends emerge, aiding in the development of tailored strategies.[414]

2. **Customized Approaches:** Armed with this knowledge, biohackers can craft personalized approaches to mental wellbeing. Whether it's managing stress, enhancing focus, or fostering emotional resilience, strategies are fine-tuned to match specific needs.[415]

---

[412] Moore, N. C. (2000). A review of EEG biofeedback treatment of anxiety disorders. Clinical Electroencephalography, 31(1), 1-6.

[413] Angelakis, E., Stathopoulou, S., Frymiare, J. L., Green, D. L., Lubar, J. F., & Kounios, J. (2007). EEG neurofeedback: A comprehensive review on system design, methodology and clinical applications. Biological Psychology, 82(1), 1-11.

[414] Trudeau, D. L. (2005). Applicability of brain wave biofeedback to substance use disorder in adolescents. Child and Adolescent Psychiatric Clinics, 14(1), 125-136.

[415] Vernon, D., Frick, A., & Gruzelier, J. H. (2004). Neurofeedback as a treatment for ADHD: A methodological review with implications for future research. Journal of Neurotherapy, 8(2), 53-82.

The Biohacker's Path to Mental Mastery

Biofeedback and neurofeedback represent cutting-edge tools that biohackers employ to track, understand, and optimize their mental and emotional states. By leveraging these technologies, individuals gain control over their physiology and brain function, making it possible to develop highly personalized strategies for mental well-being. In the quest for mental mastery, biohackers harness the power of data to thrive in an ever-demanding world.

Psychedelics as Medicine: Unveiling the Science and Potential

A Paradigm Shift

The resurgence of interest in psychedelics has opened up new possibilities for mental health biohacking. We examine the science behind psychedelics like psilocybin and MDMA, and their potential role in treating conditions such as depression, PTSD, and anxiety.

The Science of Psychedelics

1. **Psilocybin – The Magic of Mushrooms:** Psilocybin, a naturally occurring compound found in certain mushrooms, acts as a serotonin receptor agonist. This means it can profoundly alter consciousness, leading to experiences of heightened perception, introspection, and even transcendence.[416]

2. **MDMA – Beyond the Party Scene:** Often associated with recreational use, MDMA's therapeutic potential is now

---

[416] Carhart-Harris, R. L., & Goodwin, G. M. (2017). The therapeutic potential of psychedelic drugs: Past, present, and future. Neuropsychopharmacology, 42(11), 2105-2113.

gaining recognition. It enhances the release of neurotransmitters, especially serotonin, fostering feelings of empathy, emotional openness, and a profound sense of connection.[417]

Psychedelics in Mental Health Treatment

1. **Depression: Illuminating the Inner World:** Psilocybin-assisted therapy for depression has yielded groundbreaking results. Research suggests that a single guided psychedelic experience can bring about long-lasting improvements in mood and a transformative shift in one's perspective on life.[418]

2. **PTSD: Rewriting Traumatic Narratives:** MDMA-assisted psychotherapy has shown remarkable promise in treating PTSD. The substance facilitates the revisiting of traumatic memories within a controlled and supportive environment, enabling individuals to confront and process their trauma.[419]

3. **Anxiety: Dissolving the Ego:** Psychedelics, when administered under therapeutic guidance, have the potential to dissolve the rigid structures of ego and anxiety. They promote a profound sense of interconnectedness and self-acceptance, offering hope to those grappling with anxiety disorders.[420]

---

[417] Mithoefer, M. C., & Wagner, M. T. (2010). The use of MDMA in psychotherapy. PTSD Research Quarterly, 21(1), 1-7.

[418] Carhart-Harris, R. L., et al. (2016). Psilocybin with psychological support for treatment-resistant depression: An open-label feasibility study. The Lancet Psychiatry, 3(7), 619-627.

[419] Mithoefer, M. C., et al. (2018). MDMA-assisted therapy for treatment of PTSD: Study design and rationale for phase 3 trials based on pooled analysis of six phase 2 randomized controlled trials. Psychopharmacology, 235(11), 1-20.

[420] Griffiths, R. R., Johnson, M. W., Carducci, M. A., Umbricht, A., Richards, W. A., Richards, B. D., ... & Klinedinst, M. A. (2016). Psilocybin produces substantial and sustained decreases in depression and anxiety in patients with life-threatening cancer: A randomized double-blind trial. Journal of Psychopharmacology, 30(12), 1181-1197.

The Role of Set and Setting

1. **Set – The Mindset:** The individual's mindset and intentions play a pivotal role in shaping the psychedelic experience. Biohackers and therapists emphasize the importance of preparing the mind, setting intentions, and cultivating a receptive mental state.

2. **Setting – The Environment:** Equally critical is the physical and social environment in which the psychedelic journey unfolds. Controlled and supportive settings, often in therapeutic or ceremonial contexts, maximize the potential for positive outcomes.

Challenges and Future Directions

1. **Safety Concerns:** It's important to acknowledge that psychedelics are not without risks. Proper dosing, screening for contraindications, and ensuring a safe environment are paramount considerations.

2. **Legal and Regulatory Hurdles:** The legal status of psychedelics varies across regions, presenting obstacles to their widespread use in therapeutic settings. However, evolving research and changing perceptions are gradually reshaping the landscape.

A Promising Frontier in Mental Health

The science behind psychedelics, including psilocybin and MDMA, is illuminating new pathways toward treating mental health conditions that have long resisted conventional therapies. Biohackers and therapists alike approach these substances with cautious optimism, recognizing their potential to offer profound healing experiences when used responsibly and under the guidance of trained professionals. As we journey forward, the transformative power of psychedelics in mental health treatment promises to be a compelling story of hope and healing.

Psychedelic-Assisted Therapy: A Paradigm Shift in Mental Health

In the emerging field of psychedelic-assisted therapy, these substances are used in a therapeutic context under the guidance of trained professionals. The promises and challenges of this approach and its potential to transform mental health treatment are discussed below.

The Promise of Psychedelic-Assisted Therapy

1. **Reconnecting with Psychedelics:** Psychedelic-assisted therapy marks a reconnection with substances that have been used by various cultures for millennia in ceremonial and healing rituals. It acknowledges their profound potential for mental and emotional healing.

2. **Addressing Treatment-Resistant Conditions:** Traditional therapies often fall short in addressing treatment-resistant conditions such as severe depression, PTSD, and anxiety disorders. Psychedelics offer new hope for those who have exhausted conventional treatment options.

3. **Rapid and Lasting Transformation:** Studies have shown that a single guided psychedelic experience can lead to profound and enduring changes in a person's mental state, providing a unique opportunity for rapid transformation.[421]

Challenges and Considerations

1. **Safety and Legal Complexities:** The therapeutic use of psychedelics raises safety concerns, including the risk

---

[421] Carhart-Harris, R. L., et al. (2016). Psilocybin with psychological support for treatment-resistant depression: An open-label feasibility study. The Lancet Psychiatry, 3(7), 619-627; Mithoefer, M. C., et al. (2018). MDMA-assisted therapy for treatment of PTSD: Study design and rationale for phase 3 trials based on pooled analysis of six phase 2 randomized controlled trials. Psychopharmacology, 235(11), 1-20.

of adverse reactions. Furthermore, the legal status of these substances varies widely, posing regulatory challenges that researchers and practitioners must navigate.

2. **Need for Specialized Training:** Psychedelic-assisted therapy demands specialized training for therapists. These professionals must be well-versed in the unique dynamics of psychedelic experiences and be equipped to provide the necessary support and guidance.

3. **Integration and Aftercare:** The integration of psychedelic experiences into daily life is a crucial aspect of therapy. Ensuring that patients receive appropriate aftercare and support is vital for maximizing the benefits and minimizing potential risks.

Transforming Mental Health Treatment

1. **Exploring New Horizons:** Psychedelic-assisted therapy is pushing the boundaries of what's possible in mental health treatment. It offers a promising alternative for individuals who have found little relief through traditional approaches.

2. **Holistic Healing:** By addressing the symptoms and underlying causes of mental health conditions, this approach offers a more holistic form of healing. It encourages individuals to confront their traumas, gain insights, and embark on a path of self-discovery and growth.

3. **Opening the Door to Research:** The resurgence of interest in psychedelics has sparked a wave of research, shedding light on the neuroscience of these substances and their therapeutic potential. This research may lead to even more innovative and effective treatments in the future.

A Bright Future Beckons

Psychedelic-assisted therapy represents a remarkable paradigm shift in mental health treatment. It holds the promise of providing relief to individuals who have long suffered in silence, offering them the opportunity for profound transformation and healing. While challenges and complexities abound, the growing acceptance and exploration of this approach give rise to a hopeful future where mental health care is more compassionate, holistic, and effective.

The Power of Community: Nurturing Mental Wellbeing Through Connection

Loneliness and Isolation

Social isolation and loneliness are pervasive issues that can negatively impact mental health. The importance of building and maintaining meaningful relationships cannot be overstated.

The Human Need for Connection

1. **Wired for Connection:** Humans are inherently social beings. Our brains are wired for connection, and our wellbeing is intricately linked to the quality of our relationships. Meaningful social bonds are essential for our mental health.[422]

2. **The Loneliness Epidemic:** In an age of digital connectivity, loneliness has become an epidemic. Paradoxically, while we have more ways to connect than ever before, genuine human connection seems scarcer. Loneliness can lead to a range of mental health issues, including depression and anxiety.[423]

---

[422] Baumeister, R. F., & Leary, M. R. (1995). The need to belong: Desire for interpersonal attachments as a fundamental human motivation. Psychological Bulletin, 117(3), 497–529.

[423] Cacioppo, J. T., & Patrick, W. (2008). Loneliness: Human Nature and the Need for Social Connection. W. W. Norton & Company.

Community As a Source of Support

1. **Emotional Resilience:** Community provides a support system during times of crisis or emotional distress. Knowing that we have people who care about us and are willing to listen and offer support can enhance our emotional resilience.

2. **Shared Experiences:** Communities often share common experiences and challenges. This sense of belonging and shared understanding can alleviate feelings of isolation and help individuals navigate life's ups and downs more effectively.

Positive Social Interactions and Mental Health

1. **The Hormonal Influence:** Positive social interactions trigger the release of oxytocin and endorphins, often referred to as "feel-good" hormones. These neurochemical responses promote a sense of wellbeing and happiness.[424]

2. **Stress Buffer:** Meaningful social connections act as a buffer against stress. Having a community to turn to during stressful times can mitigate the harmful effects of chronic stress on mental health.[425]

Community Building and Mental Wellbeing

1. **Active Engagement:** Building and maintaining community requires active engagement. This might involve joining clubs, volunteering, participating in group activities, or simply reaching out to friends and neighbors.

2. **Technology's Role:** While technology can sometimes contribute to feelings of isolation, it can also be a tool for

---

[424] Carter, C. S. (1998). Neuroendocrine perspectives on social attachment and love. Psychoneuroendocrinology, 23(8), 779-818.

[425] Cohen, S. (2004). Social relationships and health. American Psychologist, 59(8), 676-684.

community building. Online support groups and social networks can connect people with shared interests or challenges, engendering a sense of community.

The Healing Power of Connection

Community is not just a collection of people; it's a source of healing, support, and belonging. As you navigate the complexities of modern life, the importance of nurturing meaningful relationships and developing a sense of community cannot be overstated. In a world where isolation and loneliness are on the rise, we must recognize the vital role that genuine human connection plays in our mental well-being. Together, we can build communities that nurture our souls, enrich our lives, and provide a solid foundation for mental health and resilience.

The Invaluable Role of Supportive Communities: Fostering Encouragement, Accountability, and Belonging

Biohackers recognize that they are not alone in their journey toward optimal mental health. This is where the value of a supportive community, in-person or online, and how it can provide encouragement, accountability, and a sense of belonging, is a key consideration.

The Essence of Supportive Communities

A. **Encouragement:** Supportive communities serve as incubators of encouragement. They offer a nurturing environment where individuals can share their goals, dreams, and aspirations. Here, members often find the motivation they need to pursue their passions and overcome challenges.[426]

---

[426] Deci, E. L., & Ryan, R. M. (1985). Intrinsic Motivation and Self-Determination in Human Behavior. Springer Science & Business Media.

B. **Accountability:** Within a community, accountability flourishes. Members commit to their goals, and the collective expectation of progress serves as a powerful driving force. Accountability partners or mentors can help individuals stay on track, celebrate victories, and learn from setbacks.[427]

A Sense of Belonging

A. **Human Connection:** In a world often characterized by digital isolation, the importance of genuine human connection cannot be overstated. Supportive communities offer a space where individuals can relate to one another, share experiences, and truly belong.[428]

B. **Shared Values:** These communities often revolve around shared values or interests. This common ground not only fosters a sense of belonging but also enables members to tap into collective wisdom, creativity, and passion.

In-Person vs. Online Communities

A. **In-Person Communities:** Face-to-face interactions in local communities or organizations offer the benefits of physical presence and direct engagement. They can be particularly effective for building deep, lasting connections.

B. **Online Communities:** The digital realm has opened up a vast landscape of online communities, ranging from social media groups to specialized forums. These spaces provide convenience and accessibility, making it easier for individuals to connect with like-minded people worldwide.

---

[427] Gollwitzer, P. M. (1999). Implementation intentions: Strong effects of simple plans. American Psychologist, 54(7), 493-503.

[428] Baumeister, R. F., & Leary, M. R. (1995). The need to belong: Desire for interpersonal attachments as a fundamental human motivation. Psychological Bulletin, 117(3), 497-529.

Examples of Supportive Communities

A. **Fitness and Wellness Groups:** Whether at the gym, in yoga studios, or within virtual fitness challenges, these communities encourage individuals to lead healthier lives by sharing workouts, recipes, and progress.

B. **Professional Networks:** Networking groups, both in-person and on platforms like LinkedIn, empower individuals to advance in their careers, seek mentorship, and exchange industry insights.

C. **Mental Health Support:** Online forums and local support groups provide solace and guidance for those navigating mental health challenges. These communities reduce stigma and offer empathy and coping strategies.

The Transformative Power of Support

Supportive communities are more than just gatherings of people—they are catalysts for personal growth and fulfillment. Through encouragement, accountability, and a profound sense of belonging, these communities empower you to pursue your dreams, overcome obstacles, and find meaning in your journeys.

Biohacking for mental health encompasses a wide range of strategies and techniques, from stress management and biofeedback to the potential benefits of psychedelics and the vital role of community and connection. By taking a holistic approach to mental wellbeing that includes all of these facets, biohackers strive to optimize their cognitive and emotional states, ultimately leading to a happier, more fulfilling life.

CHAPTER 10

TRACKING AND SELF-EXPERIMENTATION

Data is the lifeblood of biohacking. In this chapter, we explore the significance of data collection and its role in the biohacking journey. From the tools and technologies used for tracking to the art of designing personal experiments and analyzing the results, this chapter dives into the world of self-experimentation and data-driven optimization.

The Importance of Data Collection

Harnessing the Power of Data: Transforming Health, Performance, and Wellbeing

Biohackers understand that data is the foundation of their journey. Collecting data on various aspects of health, performance, and wellbeing is crucial for making informed decisions and tracking progress. Underscoring this importance is the setting of clear goals and objectives to guide data collection efforts.

The Data-Driven Journey

A. **Informed Decision-Making:** Data collection serves as the compass on your biohacking journey. It empowers you to make informed decisions by providing insights into your body's responses, strengths, and areas that need improvement.

B. **Personalized Optimization:** Every individual is unique, and data collection allows for personalized optimization. By tracking specific metrics, you can tailor your biohacking strategies to align with your goals and address your unique needs.[429]

Setting Clear Goals and Objectives

A. **Defining Success:** Clear, well-defined goals serve as the foundation of effective data collection. Whether it's achieving a certain fitness level, improving sleep quality, or enhancing cognitive performance, setting clear objectives helps you focus your efforts.

B. **Measurable Outcomes:** Goals should be accompanied by measurable outcomes. These metrics could include physical measurements, biomarkers, or specific performance benchmarks. Measurable outcomes provide a tangible way to assess progress.[430]

Key Aspects of Data Collection

A. **Health Metrics:** Monitoring vital signs, blood pressure, heart rate, and biomarkers such as cholesterol levels can provide valuable insights into your overall health and help identify potential health risks.

---

[429] Doherty, A., & Higham, D. (2019). Personalized and data-driven cognitive modeling. Frontiers in Psychology, 10, 367.

[430] Locke, E. A., & Latham, G. P. (2002). Building a practically useful theory of goal setting and task motivation: A 35-year odyssey. American Psychologist, 57(9), 705-717.

B. **Performance Metrics:** Athletes and individuals seeking performance improvement often track metrics such as strength, endurance, speed, and agility. These metrics can inform training programs and guide performance enhancement.

C. **Wellbeing Metrics:** Psychological wellbeing is equally important. Collecting data on mood, stress levels, sleep quality, and cognitive function allows you to identify patterns and make adjustments for better mental health.[431]

Tools and Technologies for Data Collection

A. **Wearables:** Fitness trackers, smartwatches, and health monitoring devices provide real-time data on physical activity, sleep, heart rate, and more.

B. **Apps and Software:** Mobile apps and software platforms offer a convenient way to log and analyze data, from food intake to workout routines to sleep patterns.

C. **Lab Tests:** Periodic lab tests conducted by healthcare professionals can provide in-depth insights into various biomarkers and health indicators.

Data Interpretation and Action

A. **Analyzing Trends:** Collecting data is only half the equation. The other half is analyzing the trends and patterns within the data. This analysis guides your decision-making process.

B. **Iterative Improvement:** Armed with insights from data, you can iterate on your biohacking strategies. Whether it's

---

[431] Diener, E., Emmons, R. A., Larsen, R. J., & Griffin, S. (1985). The satisfaction with life scale. Journal of Personality Assessment, 49(1), 71-75.

adjusting your diet, modifying your exercise routine, or fine-tuning your sleep habits, data helps you refine your approach.[432]

Empowering Your Biohacking Journey

Data collection is the backbone of biohacking, providing the information needed to make informed decisions and drive progress. By setting clear goals and objectives, choosing the right metrics to track, and leveraging tools and technologies, you can harness the power of data to optimize your health, enhance your performance, and elevate your overall wellbeing.

The Multifaceted World of Biohacking Data: Illuminating Your Biohacking Journey

Data comes in many forms, including physiological measurements (e.g., heart rate, blood pressure), biomarker data (e.g., blood tests, genetic data), and subjective data (e.g., mood, sleep quality). We explore the different types of data biohackers collect and how each contributes to a comprehensive understanding of one's biohacking journey.

Physical Health Data

    A. **Vital Signs:** Biohackers monitor vital signs such as heart rate, blood pressure, and body temperature to assess their overall health. Fluctuations in these metrics can signal potential issues or improvements.

    B. **Biomarkers:** Regular blood tests reveal critical information about metabolic health, cholesterol levels, hormone balance, and more. These biomarkers offer insights into the body's internal workings.

---

[432] Landers, D. M., & Arent, S. M. (2007). Physical activity and mental health. In G. Tenenbaum & R. C. Eklund (Eds.), Handbook of Sport Psychology (pp. 469-491). John Wiley & Sons.

C. **Body Composition:** Tracking body fat percentage, muscle mass, and weight provides a comprehensive view of physical changes resulting from diet, exercise, and lifestyle modifications.

Performance Metrics

A. **Fitness Data:** Athletes and fitness enthusiasts collect data on strength, endurance, speed, and flexibility to optimize training routines and track progress.

B. **Cognitive Metrics:** Cognitive performance data, including memory, reaction time, and concentration, aid in assessing the impact of lifestyle choices on mental acuity.

Nutritional Data

A. **Dietary Intake:** Detailed records of food and drink consumption help biohackers assess nutritional intake, identify dietary patterns, and make informed adjustments to optimize health and energy levels.

B. **Nutrient Tracking:** Biohackers often delve deeper into nutrient tracking, monitoring the intake of specific vitamins, minerals, and macronutrients to address deficiencies and achieve optimal nutrition.

Sleep and Wellbeing Data

A. **Sleep Patterns:** Sleep tracking data, including sleep duration and quality, reveal crucial insights into restorative sleep. Disruptions in sleep can impact mood, cognitive function, and wellbeing.

B. **Psychological Metrics:** Collecting data on mood, stress levels, and emotional wellbeing contributes to a comprehensive understanding of mental health and highlights areas for improvement.

Environmental and Lifestyle Data

    A. **Environmental Factors:** Data on exposure to environmental toxins, air quality, and radiation levels contribute to understanding how the surrounding environment impacts health.

    B. **Activity and Habits:** Tracking daily habits, including exercise routines, meditation practices, and exposure to natural light, provides valuable context for assessing wellbeing.

Genetic and Epigenetic Data

    A. **Genetic Testing:** Some biohackers opt for genetic testing to gain insights into their genetic predispositions, helping them tailor lifestyle choices and interventions accordingly.

    B. **Epigenetic Changes:** Monitoring epigenetic modifications offers a dynamic view of how lifestyle changes impact gene expression and long-term health.

Wearables and Technology

    A. **Wearable Devices:** Smartwatches, fitness trackers, and health apps collect real-time data on physical activity, sleep, and other vital signs, providing continuous insights.

    B. **Quantified Self Tools:** Biohackers leverage an array of quantified self-tools to automate data collection and analysis, streamlining their tracking efforts.

Integration and Insights

Biohackers recognize that the integration and analysis of diverse data types are essential for deriving meaningful insights. By combining and interpreting these multidimensional datasets, individuals can tailor their biohacking strategies, making informed decisions to optimize their health, performance, and wellbeing.

The Tapestry of Data in Biohacking

The multifaceted world of biohacking data weaves together physical health, performance, nutrition, sleep, wellbeing, genetics, lifestyle, and technology. By collecting and integrating these diverse data types, biohackers gain a holistic view of their biohacking journey, empowering them to make informed choices and achieve their goals.

Biohacking Tools and Technologies

Biohacking Gadgets and Tools: Empowering Self-Experimentation

Biohackers leverage a wide array of tools and technologies to collect data and optimize their health. Wearable devices like fitness trackers, smartwatches, and sleep monitors, as well as lab tests, genetic testing kits, and other biohacking gadgets, can provide valuable data for self-experimentation.

Wearable Devices: A Window to Your Health

A. **Fitness Trackers:** Wearable fitness trackers, such as Fitbit and Garmin, monitor physical activity, heart rate, and sleep patterns. They offer real-time insights into daily steps, exercise intensity, and sleep quality, enabling users to adjust their routines for better health and performance.[433]

B. **Smartwatches:** Smartwatches like the Apple Watch and Samsung Galaxy Watch extend beyond fitness tracking. They provide a holistic view of health by integrating features like ECG monitoring, stress tracking, and sleep analysis, offering a 360-degree perspective on wellbeing.[434]

---

[433] Cadmus-Bertram, L. A., et al. (2015). Use of the Fitbit to measure adherence to a physical activity intervention among overweight or obese, postmenopausal women: Self-monitoring trajectory during 16 weeks. JMIR mHealth and uHealth, 3(4), e96.

[434] Apple. (2022). Apple Watch. Retrieved from https://www.apple.com/apple-watch-series-7/

C. **Sleep Monitors:** Specialized sleep-tracking wearables, like the Oura Ring and the Withings Sleep Analyzer, focus on optimizing sleep. They measure sleep stages, interruptions, and trends, helping users make data-driven adjustments to their sleep habits.[435]

Lab Tests: Illuminating the Internal Landscape

A. **Blood Panels:** Routine blood tests, conducted in collaboration with healthcare professionals, offer insights into critical biomarkers such as cholesterol levels, blood sugar, and hormone balance. These tests are essential for diagnosing health conditions and guiding interventions.[436]

B. **Advanced Biomarker Testing:** Specialized labs and services, like InsideTracker and WellnessFX, provide comprehensive biomarker analysis, offering tailored recommendations for diet, exercise, and supplementation based on individual profiles.[437]

Genetic Testing Kits: Unveiling Your DNA's Secrets

A. **Direct-to-Consumer Genetic Testing:** Services like 23andMe and AncestryDNA provide genetic insights into ancestry, traits, and health predispositions. This information empowers biohackers to make personalized choices related to nutrition, fitness, and lifestyle.[438]

B. **Genetic Wellness Platforms:** Platforms such as DNAfit and GenoPalate offer in-depth genetic analysis tailored to

---

[435] Oura Ring. (2022). The world's most advanced wearable. Retrieved from https://ouraring.com/

[436] American Heart Association. (2017). Understanding your cholesterol levels. Retrieved from https://www.heart.org/en/health-topics/cholesterol/about-cholesterol/understanding-cholesterol-levels

[437] InsideTracker. (2022). Personalized nutrition and wellness. Retrieved from https://www.insidetracker.com/

[438] 23andMe. (2022). DNA genetic testing & analysis. Retrieved from https://www.23andme.com/

health and fitness. They provide actionable recommendations to optimize nutrition, exercise, and overall wellbeing.[439]

Other Biohacking Gadgets: Expanding Possibilities

A. **Biofeedback Devices:** Devices like heart rate variability (HRV) monitors and neurofeedback tools enable users to track and improve physiological responses to stress. Biofeedback empowers individuals to enhance mental resilience and wellbeing.[440]

B. **Environmental Sensors:** Smart home sensors and devices like the Awair air quality monitor detect environmental factors that impact health. They help biohackers optimize their living spaces for cleaner air, better lighting, and reduced exposure to toxins.[441]

Integration and Self-Experimentation

Biohackers leverage these gadgets and tools to collect a wealth of data, creating a personalized feedback loop for self-experimentation. By integrating information from wearables, lab tests, genetic insights, and more, individuals can fine-tune their diets, exercise routines, and lifestyles with precision.[442]

The Technological Frontier of Self-Optimization

Biohacking gadgets and tools represent the forefront of self-optimization. These devices offer actionable data that empower you to take

---

439 DNAfit. (2022). Unlock your full potential with DNAfit. Retrieved from https://www.dnafit.com/

440 Thoma, M.V., et al. (2018). The effect of music on the human stress response. PLoS ONE, 13(9), e0207366.

441 Awair. (2022). Awair. Retrieved from https://www.getawair.com/

442 Asprey, D. (2019). Super Human: The Bulletproof Plan to Age Backward and Maybe Even Live Forever. Harper Wave.

charge of your health. As technology continues to evolve, biohackers have an ever-expanding toolkit at their disposal, fueling the journey toward a healthier, more optimized future.

Biohacking Apps and Platforms: Unleashing the Power of Data-Driven Optimization

Modern technology has enabled biohackers to gain real-time insights into their health and performance. We explore how biohacking apps and platforms collect and analyze data, providing actionable insights and recommendations. Biohackers use these tools to monitor progress, identify trends, and make data-driven adjustments to their routines.

Data Collection: The Foundation of Biohacking Apps

Biohacking apps and platforms serve as hubs for data collection and aggregating information from various sources, including wearables, self-reports, and external databases. This data can encompass a wide range of metrics, from physical activity and sleep patterns to dietary habits and genetic information.[443]

Data Analysis: Uncovering Insights

1. **Machine Learning and AI:** Many biohacking apps employ machine learning and artificial intelligence (AI) algorithms to analyze the collected data. These sophisticated tools can identify patterns, correlations, and anomalies that may not be apparent through manual analysis.

2. **Trend Identification:** Biohacking platforms excel at identifying trends within the data. For example, they can detect

---

[443] Chen, Y., & Saini, R. (2021). Machine learning applications in bioinformatics. In Machine Learning and Artificial Intelligence for Bioinformatics (pp. 3-11). Springer.

how certain dietary choices affect sleep quality or how specific exercise routines impact cognitive performance.[444]

Actionable Insights: Empowering Change

1. **Personalized Recommendations:** Based on data analysis, biohacking apps generate personalized recommendations.
   These can include dietary adjustments, exercise modifications,
   sleep hygiene practices, and supplementation plans tailored to
   an individual's unique needs and goals.[445]

2. **Goal Setting:** Biohackers can set specific goals within these
   platforms, and the apps provide guidance on how to achieve
   them. Whether it's weight loss, muscle gain, or better sleep,
   the apps offer step-by-step plans.

3. **Tracking Progress:** Biohacking apps offer visual represen-
   tations of progress, allowing users to see how their metrics
   change over time. This visual feedback reinforces positive
   habits and motivates continued optimization.

Integration and Holistic Insights

Biohacking apps often provide a holistic view of wellbeing by integrating data from various aspects of life, such as physical health, nutrition, sleep, and stress management. This comprehensive approach
allows users to see how different factors interrelate and influence
overall health and performance.[446]

---

[444] Perna, G., et al. (2018). Artificial intelligence, natural language processing, and machine
learning applications to vascular and interventional radiology. European Radiology Experimental, 2(1), 28.

[445] Shuren, J. (2019). Artificial Intelligence and Machine Learning in Software as a Medical
Device. US Food and Drug Administration.

[446] Hood, L., & Flores, M. (2012). A personal view on systems medicine and the emergence
of proactive P4 medicine: Predictive, preventive, personalized and participatory. New Bio-
technology, 29(6), 613-624.

User Empowerment: Making Informed Decisions

A. **Data Ownership:** Many biohacking apps emphasize user ownership of data. This means individuals have control over their information and can choose to share it with healthcare professionals or researchers for further analysis.

B. **Continuous Learning:** Biohacking platforms often offer educational content, ensuring that users understand the significance of their data and the rationale behind recommended changes.[447]

The Future of Personalized Optimization

Biohacking apps and platforms represent the future of personalized optimization. By harnessing the power of data collection, analysis, and actionable insights, biohackers can make informed decisions that propel them toward their health and performance goals. As technology advances, these tools will play an increasingly vital role in the pursuit of wellbeing.

Designing Personal Experiments: The Art and Science of Biohacking Hypotheses

The Art of Experimentation

Self-experimentation is at the heart of biohacking. We delve into the principles of designing personal experiments, including formulating hypotheses, defining variables, and setting clear objectives. Biohackers learn to create structured experiments that yield meaningful results.

The Scientific Approach to Biohacking

A. **Formulating Hypotheses:** At the heart of any experiment lies a well-crafted hypothesis—a testable statement that

---

[447] Patel, V. L., et al. (2018). Ten common mistakes in conducting usability studies. Handbook of Human Factors and Ergonomics in Health Care and Patient Safety, 465-475.

predicts a relationship between variables. Hypotheses in bio-hacking are often inspired by specific goals. For example, if your objective is to improve sleep quality, your hypothesis might be: "Increasing daily exposure to natural light will lead to better sleep."

B. **Defining Variables:** Variables are factors that can change in an experiment. In biohacking, there are independent variables (those you manipulate, like the amount of exercise) and dependent variables (those you measure, like changes in heart rate). By clearly defining variables, you ensure your experiment is focused and controlled.

Setting Clear Objectives: The Why and What of Your Experiment

A. **Why Are You Experimenting?** Begin by defining your overarching goal. Is it to enhance cognitive function, optimize nutrition, or increase physical endurance? Understanding your purpose will guide your experiment's design and ensure it remains relevant to your biohacking journey.

B. **What Will You Measure?** Identify the specific metrics or outcomes you'll use to evaluate the success of your experiment. These could include biomarkers, performance indicators, or self-reported data like mood and sleep quality.[448]

Experiment Design: From Control Groups to Baseline Data

A. **Control Groups:** In some biohacking experiments, it's valuable to have a control group—a group that doesn't undergo the intervention. This allows you to compare results and determine if the changes observed are due to your biohacking efforts or unrelated factors.

---

[448] Lakens, D. (2013). Calculating and reporting effect sizes to facilitate cumulative science: A practical primer for t-tests and ANOVAs. Frontiers in Psychology, 4, 863.

B. **Baseline Data:** Collect baseline data before implementing any changes. Baseline data provide a reference point against which you can measure the impact of your biohacking interventions. For example, if you want to assess the effects of a new diet plan on cholesterol levels, measure your cholesterol before starting the diet.

Ethical Considerations and Safety

A. **Ethical Research:** Conduct your personal experiments with ethical considerations in mind. Ensure your experiments do not harm your health or wellbeing, and respect privacy and consent if you involve others in your research.

B. **Safety First:** Prioritize safety in your experiments. Avoid risky behaviors or interventions that could have adverse effects on your health.

Iterative Learning and Adaptation

A. **Data Collection:** Throughout your experiment, collect data diligently. Use tools and methods, such as biohacking apps and wearables, to capture relevant information accurately.

B. **Analysis and Reflection:** After the experiment, analyze your data and reflect on the results. Did your hypothesis hold true? What can you learn from the data? Use your findings to adjust your biohacking strategies for continuous improvement.[449]

The Path to Informed Biohacking

Designing personal experiments is both an art and a science. By formulating hypotheses, defining variables, and setting clear objectives,

---

[449] Thiese, M. S. (2014). Observational and interventional study design types; An overview. Biochemia Medica, 24(2), 199-210.

biohackers embark on a journey of self-discovery and optimization. Ethical considerations and a commitment to safety ensure that biohacking experiments contribute to personal growth and wellbeing.

Ethical Considerations in Biohacking: Navigating the Path to Responsible Self-Experimentation

Practical guidance on how to conduct experiments safely and ethically, including considerations such as data integrity, ethical dilemmas, and the importance of informed consent, is important for anyone on this path. Biohackers understand the responsibility of conducting experiments that contribute positively to their wellbeing.

Data Integrity: The Cornerstone of Ethical Biohacking

A. **Accurate Data Collection:** Maintaining data integrity is paramount in biohacking. Accurate and honest data collection ensures that the results of your experiments are reliable and trustworthy.

B. **Transparency in Reporting:** Transparently report all results, even if they do not align with your expectations. This fosters trust in the biohacking community and allows others to learn from your experiences.

Informed Consent: Respecting Autonomy

A. **Self-Consent:** As a biohacker, you are both the experimenter and the subject. While you don't need external consent, it's essential to obtain your informed self-consent before initiating any experiment. Clearly understand the risks and potential outcomes.

B. **Involving Others:** If your biohacking experiments involve others, ensure they provide informed consent. They should be aware of the purpose of the experiment, potential risks, and their right to withdraw at any time.

Respect for Privacy: Safeguarding Personal Data

A. **Data Privacy:** Safeguard your personal data and sensitive health information. Use secure platforms and devices for data collection and be mindful of sharing your data only with trusted sources.

B. **Anonymity and Pseudonymity:** When sharing your biohacking experiences or data with the community, consider using pseudonyms or anonymous profiles to protect your privacy.[450]

Ethical Dilemmas: Balancing Exploration and Responsibility

A. **Risk-Benefit Analysis:** Before embarking on an experiment, conduct a thorough risk-benefit analysis. Consider the potential benefits against the risks involved. Avoid experiments with disproportionately high risks and limited benefits.

B. **Unintended Consequences:** Anticipate and mitigate unintended consequences of your experiments. Be prepared to adapt or halt an experiment if unforeseen issues arise.

Openness and Collaboration: Fostering Ethical Biohacking Communities

A. **Sharing Knowledge:** Share your biohacking knowledge and experiences with others openly and responsibly. This fosters a collaborative and supportive biohacking community.

B. **Community Guidelines:** Participate in or establish community guidelines that emphasize ethical conduct, respect, and responsible experimentation. Encourage peer review and constructive feedback.

---

[450] Moorhead, S. A., et al. (2013). A new dimension of health care: Systematic review of the uses, benefits, and limitations of social media for health communication. Journal of Medical Internet Research, 15(4), e85.

The Biohacker's Ethical Responsibility

Biohackers understand that with great autonomy comes great responsibility. By upholding principles of data integrity, informed consent, privacy, and ethical conduct, biohackers can ensure that their experiments contribute positively to their wellbeing and the broader biohacking community.[451]

The Feedback Loop: Biohacking's Engine of Continuous Improvement

The Data Feedback Loop

Collecting data is only the first step. We explore how biohackers analyze their data, identifying patterns, correlations, and outliers. The chapter discusses the importance of maintaining a feedback loop between data analysis and biohacking strategies, allowing for continuous adjustment and optimization.

The Feedback Loop: An Iterative Journey

A. **Data Collection and Analysis:** The feedback loop begins with data collection and rigorous analysis. Biohackers gather information from various sources, including wearables, lab tests, and self-reports. Advanced tools, such as biohacking apps and platforms, aid in data interpretation.

B. **Identification of Trends and Patterns:** Through data analysis, biohackers identify trends, patterns, and correlations within their datasets. For instance, they may discover how dietary changes affect mood or how exercise impacts sleep quality.

---

[451] Ross, S. E., & Lin, C. T. (2003). The effects of promoting patient access to medical records: A review. Journal of the American Medical Informatics Association, 10(2), 129-138.

Continuous Adjustment: Navigating the Biohacking Landscape

A. **Optimizing Interventions:** Armed with data-driven insights, biohackers make informed adjustments to their interventions. This may involve modifying dietary choices, fine-tuning exercise routines, or altering sleep hygiene practices.

B. **Setting New Goals:** Biohackers often set new goals based on their findings. For instance, if they observe that a particular dietary change positively impacts energy levels, they might set a new goal to further enhance their overall vitality.

Measurement and Evaluation: Tracking Progress

A. **Monitoring Metrics:** Biohackers continue to monitor relevant metrics and indicators throughout the adjustment phase. This ongoing measurement provides real-time feedback on the effectiveness of the changes implemented.

B. **Assessing Impact:** Assessing the impact of adjustments is a critical step. Biohackers evaluate whether the modifications have led to the desired improvements in health, performance, or wellbeing.

Iterative Learning: A Biohacker's Journey of Discovery

A. **Learning from Experience:** Biohackers view their journey as an ongoing learning experience. Each iteration of the feedback loop contributes to a deeper understanding of their body's responses and needs.

B. **Documenting Insights:** Biohackers document their insights, successes, and failures. This knowledge serves as a valuable resource for future experimentation and informs their biohacking community.

Biohacking Community: Sharing Insights and Discoveries

A. **Peer Review and Collaboration:** Biohackers often engage in peer review and collaboration within the community. Sharing experiences, results, and strategies promotes collective learning and ethical biohacking practices.

The Evolution of Self-Optimization

The feedback loop is the engine that propels biohacking forward. It embodies the essence of continuous improvement, allowing biohackers to adapt, optimize, and thrive on their journey of self-discovery and self-optimization. In this ever-evolving process, biohackers unlock their full potential for health, performance, and wellbeing.

Data-Driven Refinement: Biohackers' Journey to Goal Achievement

Biohackers embrace the idea of iterative experimentation by using data-driven insights to refine their strategies and make incremental adjustments to achieve their goals. This approach enables biohackers to adapt and evolve their routines over time.

The Power of Data-Driven Insights

A. **Collecting Rich Data:** Biohackers begin by collecting comprehensive data from various sources. This may include wearable devices, lab tests, and self-reports, all of which provide a holistic view of their current state.

B. **Data Analysis:** Through advanced tools and platforms, biohackers analyze the collected data meticulously. They identify trends, correlations, and patterns that inform their understanding of how various factors influence their wellbeing.

Setting Clear Goals

A. **Defining Objectives:** Biohackers establish clear and specific objectives that align with their broader goals. Whether it's improving cognitive performance, optimizing sleep, or enhancing physical endurance, having well-defined goals serves as a compass for their biohacking journey.

B. **Quantifying Progress:** Biohackers quantify their goals whenever possible. This allows them to track progress objectively and measure the impact of their interventions.

Incremental Adjustments

A. **Evidence-Based Changes:** Armed with data-driven insights, biohackers make evidence-based adjustments to their strategies. For example, if they aim to reduce stress, they may experiment with meditation techniques based on data suggesting its effectiveness.

B. **Gradual Modifications:** Biohackers prefer gradual modifications over radical changes. This approach allows them to assess the impact of each adjustment with precision and minimize the risk of unintended consequences.

Continuous Monitoring

A. **Real-Time Feedback:** Biohackers use ongoing data collection to gain real-time feedback on the effectiveness of their adjustments. For example, they may monitor heart rate variability (HRV) to gauge stress levels and adapt stress-reduction techniques accordingly.

B. **Regular Assessments:** Regular assessments help biohackers evaluate their progress objectively. They compare current metrics with baseline data to determine if they are moving closer to their goals.

Documenting Insights

A. **Keeping Records:** Biohackers maintain detailed records of their biohacking experiments, including the strategies implemented, changes made, and the resulting outcomes. This documentation serves as a valuable resource for future endeavors.

B. **Sharing Knowledge:** Biohackers often share their insights and experiences with the broader biohacking community. This collaborative approach fosters a culture of learning and helps others benefit from their discoveries.

Achieving Biohacking Goals

A. **Continuous Refinement:** Biohackers understand that the path to achieving their goals is an iterative process.

B. **Celebrating Success:** Along the way, biohackers celebrate their successes, no matter how small. Acknowledging achievements reinforces positive habits and maintains motivation for further progress.

A Journey of Self-Optimization

Biohackers embark on a journey of self-optimization guided by data-driven insights. By making incremental adjustments to their strategies, they inch closer to achieving their biohacking goals, all while contributing to the ever-evolving body of knowledge within the biohacking community.

Tracking and self-experimentation are the essence of biohacking. By collecting data, leveraging tools and technologies, designing personal experiments, and analyzing results, biohackers embark on a journey of continuous self-improvement and optimization.

CHAPTER 11

ETHICAL CONSIDERATIONS

I n the world of biohacking, where individuals strive to optimize their bodies and minds, ethical considerations play a vital role. This chapter explores the complex ethical dilemmas that biohackers encounter, delving into the balancing act between personal ambition and responsibility. It's about the importance of ensuring safety, obtaining informed consent, and navigating the intricate moral landscape of biohacking.

The Ethical Dilemmas in Biohacking

Playing with Boundaries

Biohacking often involves pushing the boundaries of what is considered normal or acceptable in the pursuit of self-improvement. This section examines the ethical dilemmas that arise when biohackers experiment with untested substances, technologies, or techniques. We explore the potential risks and consequences of these actions.

The Pursuit of the Unknown

A. **Biohacker's Quest:** Biohackers are known for their curiosity and willingness to explore the uncharted territories of self-improvement. They often seek innovative approaches, including emerging technologies and unconventional substances, in their quest for enhanced health and performance.

B. **Ethical Challenges:** The pursuit of the unknown introduces ethical challenges, particularly when biohackers venture into realms with limited scientific validation or clear safety profiles.

Potential Risks and Consequences

A. **Health Risks:** Uncharted biohacking experiments can carry inherent health risks. Without established safety data, biohackers may expose themselves to unforeseen dangers, ranging from mild side effects to severe health complications.

B. **Lack of Informed Consent:** In cases involving untested technologies or substances, informed consent may be compromised. Biohackers must grapple with the ethical implications of self-experimentation when they lack comprehensive knowledge about potential risks.

Ethical Considerations in Biohacking

A. **Autonomy vs. Safety:** The biohacker's autonomy to explore novel interventions must be weighed against the need for safety. Ethical biohackers strive to strike a balance that respects individual choice while minimizing harm.[452]

---

[452] Harris, J., & Savulescu, J. (2017). The ethics of human enhancement. In The Oxford Handbook of Philosophy of Technology (pp. 428-446). Oxford University Press.

B. **Transparency and Documentation:** Ethical biohackers document their experiments meticulously, including details of substances used, methodologies applied, and outcomes observed. This commitment to transparency serves to inform others and mitigate potential harm.

Community Responsibility

A. **Peer Review and Collaboration:** The biohacking community plays a pivotal role in maintaining ethical standards. Peer review and collaboration ensure that uncharted biohacking endeavors are subjected to scrutiny, reducing the likelihood of reckless experimentation.

B. **Education and Ethical Guidelines:** Ethical biohackers actively contribute to education and the development of ethical guidelines within the community. They encourage responsible experimentation and advocate for safety.

The Role of Regulatory Bodies

A. **Regulation and Oversight:** Biohackers often operate in a legal gray area, where regulations may not specifically address their activities. Ethical dilemmas may arise when biohackers navigate this regulatory landscape. They advocate for responsible regulation that strikes a balance between innovation and safety.

B. **Engagement with Authorities:** Some biohackers engage with regulatory bodies and authorities to ensure their experiments adhere to existing legal frameworks. Ethical biohackers recognize the importance of legal compliance in safeguarding both their interests and the public's wellbeing.[453]

---

[453] Bubela, T., et al. (2020). Ethical and regulatory approaches to cognitive enhancement. In The Oxford Handbook of Neuroethics (pp. 673-689). Oxford University Press.

Ethical Biohacking in Uncharted Waters

Biohackers are pioneers of self-improvement, but they must navigate ethical dilemmas when exploring untested substances, technologies, or techniques. By prioritizing safety, transparency, collaboration, and adherence to ethical guidelines, biohackers can strike a responsible balance between pushing boundaries and preserving their wellbeing.

Ethical Implications of Enhancement: Navigating Questions of Fairness and Access

Biohackers frequently seek to enhance their cognitive abilities, physical performance, and overall wellbeing. In doing so, they consider the ethical implications of pursuing enhancement, including questions of fairness, access, and the potential for creating societal disparities.

The Pursuit of Enhancement: A Moral Quandary

A. **Definition of Enhancement:** Enhancement refers to the deliberate improvement of human capacities or characteristics beyond what is considered typical or normal. Biohackers often engage in enhancement activities to achieve physical, cognitive, or sensory advancements.

B. **Ethical Questions:** The pursuit of enhancement raises complex ethical questions related to the fairness of access to these technologies, the potential creation of societal disparities, and the moral boundaries of self-improvement.

Fairness and Equity

A. **Access to Enhancement Technologies:** One of the central ethical concerns is the unequal access to enhancement technologies. High costs, limited availability, and socioeconomic disparities can create an unfair advantage for those who can afford enhancement.

B. **The "Enhancement Divide":** The emergence of an "enhancement divide" could exacerbate existing inequalities, as some individuals may gain access to enhancements while others remain excluded, potentially leading to societal fragmentation.

Societal Disparities

A. **Exacerbating Inequalities:** The pursuit of enhancement can either narrow or widen societal disparities. Ethical biohackers advocate for strategies that ensure the benefits of enhancement are distributed equitably.

B. **Psychological and Social Impacts:** The psychological and social impacts of enhancement, such as changes in self-esteem or social dynamics, may create unintended consequences that require ethical consideration.[454]

Balancing Autonomy and Societal Wellbeing

A. **Individual Autonomy:** Ethical biohackers emphasize the importance of individual autonomy—the right to make choices about one's own body and self-improvement. However, they recognize the need to balance autonomy with societal wellbeing.

B. **Ethical Regulations:** Some biohackers advocate for ethical regulations that guide the responsible use of enhancement technologies, ensuring that societal interests are not undermined.[455]

---

[454] Savulescu, J., & Persson, I. (2012). The perils of cognitive enhancement and the urgent imperative to enhance the moral character of humanity. Journal of Applied Philosophy, 29(4), 322-340.
[455] Sandberg, A. (2011). Enhancement ethics: The state of the debate. In Enhancing Human Capacities (pp. 27-45). Wiley.

Access to Enhancement Education

A. **Education and Informed Choices:** Ethical biohackers promote education and awareness to enable individuals to make informed choices regarding enhancement. They believe that access to knowledge is a fundamental aspect of fairness.

B. **Community Responsibility:** The biohacking community assumes a role in promoting ethical practices and disseminating information on enhancement. Peer review, open dialogue, and collaboration help ensure responsible enhancement pursuits.

The Ethical Tightrope of Enhancement

The pursuit of enhancement is a double-edged sword, offering immense potential for human improvement while raising significant ethical dilemmas. Biohackers navigate this tightrope by advocating for fairness, access, and the responsible use of enhancement technologies, striving to ensure that the benefits of self-improvement are shared by all.

Balancing Personal Ambition and Social Responsibility

The Drive for Self-Improvement

Biohackers are driven by a desire for self-improvement and optimization. While tension exists between personal ambition and social responsibility, biohackers balance their pursuit of individual goals with a sense of duty to the broader community.

Personal Ambition: The Drive for Self-Improvement

Personal ambition is the inner force that motivates individuals to set and achieve goals. Biohackers, driven by personal ambition, seek to optimize their health, cognitive abilities, and overall well-being. They embrace innovation, experimentation, and continuous self-improvement.

Social Responsibility: Ethical Considerations

Social responsibility calls for considering the broader impact of one's actions on society. It raises ethical questions about fairness, access to resources, and the potential consequences of personal ambition. Ethical biohackers recognize the need to balance their drive for self-improvement with a commitment to the wellbeing of others.

Finding Balance: Ethical Biohacking

Ethical biohackers navigate the tension between personal ambition and social responsibility by:

A. **Promoting Fairness:** They advocate for equitable access to self-enhancement technologies and strategies, reducing disparities between those who can and cannot afford such pursuits.

B. **Community Engagement:** Ethical biohackers actively engage with the biohacking community to foster a culture of responsible experimentation, peer review, and knowledge sharing.

C. **Regulation and Oversight:** Some biohackers support ethical regulations that guide the safe and responsible use of enhancement technologies, ensuring societal interests are not compromised.

The Harmonious Coexistence

The tension between personal ambition and social responsibility is not irreconcilable. Ethical biohackers exemplify how you can pursue self-improvement while upholding the principles of fairness, access, and ethical conduct. In finding this balance, you will strive for a harmonious coexistence of personal ambition and social responsibility, contributing positively to your own wellbeing and the greater good of society.

The Vital Role of Transparency in Biohacking: Sharing Experiences and Insights Responsibly

Accountability is a cornerstone of ethical biohacking. The importance of transparency in sharing biohacking experiences and outcomes, as well as the responsibility to disseminate knowledge and insights responsibly, cannot be overstated.

The Ethical Imperative of Transparency

A. **Openness As a Core Value:** Biohackers hold transparency as a core ethical value. They believe in sharing their biohacking journeys openly, including the strategies they employ, the outcomes they experience, and any challenges they encounter.

B. **Building Trust:** Transparency is a foundation for trust within the biohacking community. By openly sharing their experiences, biohackers build credibility and reliability, enabling others to learn from their insights.

Sharing Biohacking Experiences Responsibly

A. **Comprehensive Documentation:** Ethical biohackers maintain comprehensive records of their biohacking experiments. This documentation includes detailed information about methodologies, interventions, measurements, and outcomes.

B. **Balancing Success and Failure:** Responsible biohackers share successful outcomes and failures. This balanced approach provides a more accurate picture of the biohacking landscape and helps others avoid potential pitfalls.

Knowledge Dissemination: An Ethical Responsibility

A. **Educational Outreach:** Biohackers take on the responsibility of educating others about the principles and practices of biohacking. They recognize that knowledge dissemination is crucial for the growth and ethical conduct of the community.

B. **Empowering Informed Choices:** Transparent sharing empowers individuals to make informed choices about their own biohacking endeavors. It equips them with knowledge, enabling them to weigh the risks and benefits of different interventions.

Peer Review and Collaboration

A. **Peer Evaluation:** Ethical biohackers encourage peer review within the community. They actively seek feedback and constructive criticism from fellow biohackers, enhancing the quality and safety of their experiments.

B. **Collaborative Learning:** Collaboration is central to responsible knowledge sharing. Biohackers collaborate on projects, experiments, and research, pooling their collective expertise for the greater good.

Responsible Dissemination of Knowledge

A. **Avoiding Hype and Sensationalism:** Ethical biohackers avoid sensationalism and exaggerated claims. They understand the importance of presenting information factually and objectively.

B. **Citing Sources and References:** When sharing scientific or technical information, responsible biohackers provide proper citations and references, ensuring that others can verify and explore the sources independently.

The Legacy of Responsible Transparency

Transparency is not merely a guideline; it is the bedrock upon which ethical biohacking thrives. Responsible biohackers recognize their ethical duty to share experiences, outcomes, and knowledge transparently. By doing so, they contribute to the collective wisdom of the biohacking community, leaving behind a legacy of responsible transparency for future generations of self-optimizers.

Safety First in Biohacking: Mitigating Risks and Practicing Harm Reduction

The Primacy of Safety

Safety is paramount in the world of biohacking. As such, biohackers take measures to ensure their experiments and interventions are safe, both for themselves and for those who may seek to replicate their efforts. In doing so, they utilize risk mitigation strategies.

Safety as a Non-Negotiable Priority

A. **Ethical Imperative:** Biohackers view safety as an ethical imperative. They understand the potential risks associated with self-experimentation and the responsibility they have toward themselves and the broader community.

B. **Balancing Ambition and Prudence:** Biohackers strike a balance between their ambitious pursuit of self-improvement and the prudent consideration of potential risks. They acknowledge that safety should never be compromised for the sake of enhancement.

Risk Mitigation Strategies

A. **Comprehensive Research:** Before embarking on any biohacking journey, biohackers thoroughly research the interventions, substances, or technologies they plan to use. They gather data on safety profiles, potential side effects, and best practices.

B. **Consultation with Experts:** Biohackers seek advice from experts in relevant fields. They consult with medical professionals, scientists, and experienced biohackers to ensure they are well-informed about the risks and benefits.

Responsible Experimentation

A. **Gradual and Incremental Changes:** Biohackers prefer gradual and incremental changes rather than radical interventions. This approach allows them to assess the impact of each modification and mitigate potential risks effectively.

B. **Monitoring and Documentation:** Throughout their experiments, biohackers monitor relevant metrics and meticulously document their experiences. This data-driven approach helps them identify and address any unexpected developments promptly.

The Principle of Harm Reduction

A. **Embracing Harm Reduction:** Biohackers embrace the principles of harm reduction, a strategy aimed at minimizing the potential negative consequences of risky behaviors. They acknowledge that some level of risk may exist and take steps to reduce it.

B. **Sharing Lessons Learned:** Ethical biohackers share not only their successes but also their failures and lessons learned. This candid approach helps others avoid repeating potentially harmful mistakes.

Community Responsibility

A. **Peer Review and Collaboration:** Biohackers engage with their peers for feedback and collaboration. Peer review within the community helps identify potential safety concerns and enhances the overall quality of experimentation.

B. **Education and Mentorship:** Biohackers actively contribute to the education and mentorship of newcomers. They guide them toward responsible practices and instill a culture of safety within the biohacking community.

Ethical Biohacking with Safety at Its Core

Safety is not a peripheral consideration in biohacking. Instead, it is at the heart of responsible self-improvement. Biohackers prioritize safety by conducting thorough research, seeking expert guidance, practicing harm reduction, and sharing their experiences transparently. By doing so, they uphold their ethical responsibility to themselves and those who may embark on similar journeys.

Informed Consent in Biohacking: Balancing Ethics and Self-Experimentation

Informed consent is a fundamental ethical principle in biohacking that considers the necessity of fully disclosing risks, potential benefits, and uncertainties to participants in biohacking experiments. Further, there are challenges in obtaining informed consent in self-experimentation and the ethical responsibilities of biohackers when experimenting on others.

The Foundation of Informed Consent

A. **Definition:** Informed consent is a fundamental ethical principle that requires individuals to voluntarily and knowingly agree to participate in any medical or scientific experiment or intervention after being informed of all relevant information.

B. **Ethical Imperative:** Biohackers recognize that informed consent is not just a legal requirement but a moral obligation. It ensures that participants have autonomy over their choices and are protected from harm.

Informed Consent in Self-Experimentation

A. **Unique Challenges:** Self-experimentation presents unique challenges in obtaining informed consent. Biohackers must fully comprehend the risks and uncertainties associated with their interventions and acknowledge that their self-consent may be influenced by personal biases and motivations.

B. **Mitigating Bias:** To mitigate potential bias, biohackers often seek external input from experts or peers who can provide objective perspectives on the risks and benefits of their experiments.

Transparency and Full Disclosure

A. **Comprehensive Information:** Biohackers have an ethical responsibility to provide participants with comprehensive information about the experiment, including potential risks, benefits, uncertainties, and the nature of the intervention.

B. **Avoiding Coercion:** Participants must enter into the experiment voluntarily, without coercion or pressure. Biohackers ensure that individuals understand they can withdraw their consent at any time without consequences.

Ethical Responsibilities of Biohackers in Experimentation Involving Others

A. **Third-Party Participants:** When biohackers involve others in their experiments, they must obtain informed consent from these participants, following the same ethical principles of transparency and voluntary participation.

B. **Safety and Wellbeing:** Biohackers have a responsibility to prioritize the safety and wellbeing of participants. They should design experiments with safeguards in place to mini-mize harm.

Continuous Monitoring and Reevaluation

A. **Ongoing Informed Consent:** Biohackers acknowledge that the informed consent process is not a one-time event. They maintain open communication with participants, ensuring they stay informed about any evolving risks or benefits.

B. **Reevaluation and Adjustments:** Biohackers are open to reevaluating and adjusting experiments based on emerging data or participant feedback, with their informed consent at the forefront.

Ethical Biohacking Through Informed Consent

Informed consent is the cornerstone of ethical biohacking, whether in self-experimentation or experimentation involving others. Bio-hackers embrace the responsibility of providing transparent, com-prehensive information, allowing individuals to make autonomous choices regarding their participation. By adhering to these principles, biohackers uphold ethical standards while advancing the field of self-improvement responsibly.

Navigating Ethical Relativism in Biohacking: Embracing Cultural Sensitivity and Empathy

Ethical Relativism and Cultural Context

Ethical considerations can vary across cultures and individuals. With the concept of ethical relativism, biohackers navigate the moral land-scape in a diverse and interconnected world.

Ethical Relativism Unveiled

Ethical relativism acknowledges that cultural norms, historical context, and individual perspectives can profoundly influence what is considered morally acceptable or unacceptable. In essence, there is no one-size-fits-all moral framework that applies universally.

The Global and Interconnected Biohacking Community

Biohacking, by its very nature, transcends borders and boundaries. It's a global community where individuals from diverse cultural backgrounds come together to pursue self-improvement. Within this diverse landscape, the tenets of ethical relativism become particularly relevant.

Respecting Cultural Differences

Ethical biohackers recognize the importance of respecting cultural differences. They understand that imposing one's own cultural values or ethical frameworks onto others can be counterproductive and ethnocentric—a term used to describe the tendency to evaluate other cultures by the standards of one's own.

The Role of Cultural Sensitivity

Cultural sensitivity is the key to harmonious coexistence and ethical decision-making in the biohacking community. It entails an awareness and understanding of different cultural norms, values, and practices. Biohackers cultivate cultural sensitivity as a means of approaching ethical dilemmas with empathy and consideration for the rich tapestry of cultural diversity.

The Power of Empathy

Empathy, the ability to understand and share the feelings and perspectives of others, is a driving force behind ethical decision-making for biohackers. By actively engaging in perspective-taking, they endeavor to understand and appreciate different cultural viewpoints.

Ethical Relativism in Informed Consent

Informed consent is a critical ethical principle. Yet, biohackers recognize that informed consent must be tailored to the cultural and individual beliefs of participants. They take painstaking measures to ensure that participants fully grasp the ethical implications of their involvement within their cultural contexts.

A Tapestry of Ethical Biohacking

In a world marked by ethical relativism and cultural diversity, biohackers understand that embracing cultural sensitivity and empathy is paramount. By doing so, they navigate the intricate moral landscape of biohacking with respect for diverse perspectives. This commitment fosters an inclusive and ethical community that thrives in an interconnected world—a tapestry of ethical biohacking where differences are celebrated and individual autonomy is respected.

Ethical Philosophies in Biohacking: Navigating the Moral Landscape

Biohackers often adopt ethical frameworks to guide their actions and decisions, such as utilitarianism, deontology, and virtue ethics. The importance of continuous ethical reflection and moral growth are key.

Utilitarianism: The Pursuit of the Greatest Good

Utilitarianism is an ethical philosophy that centers on maximizing overall happiness or wellbeing. Biohackers who adopt a utilitarian perspective aim to optimize themselves and others to achieve the greatest good for the greatest number.

Ethical Implications: Utilitarian biohackers weigh the potential benefits of self-improvement interventions against their risks and costs. They prioritize interventions that promise the most significant positive impact on wellbeing.

Deontology: The Ethics of Duty and Principles

Deontology focuses on moral duties and principles that guide ethical decision-making. Biohackers who align with deontological ethics prioritize adherence to ethical rules and principles, even if the outcomes are uncertain.

Ethical Implications: Deontological biohackers rigorously evaluate the ethical principles underlying their interventions. They ensure that their pursuits align with principles such as autonomy, informed consent, and respect for people.

Virtue Ethics: Cultivating Moral Character

Virtue ethics emphasizes the cultivation of virtuous character traits. Biohackers embracing this philosophy prioritize personal development and nurturing virtuous qualities in their journey toward self-improvement.

Ethical Implications: Virtue-oriented biohackers focus on character development and the pursuit of moral virtues such as empathy, humility, and wisdom. They believe that ethical actions stem from virtuous character.

Continuous Ethical Reflection and Moral Growth

Biohackers understand that ethical philosophies provide valuable frameworks, but they also acknowledge that ethical decision-making is not static. Continuous ethical reflection and moral growth are essential aspects of biohacking practices.

Ethical Evolution: Biohackers engage in ongoing self-assessment and ethical reflection to adapt their practices as their understanding of ethics evolves.

Community Dialogue: Ethical biohackers foster open and respectful dialogue within the community, encouraging discussions about the ethical implications of emerging technologies and interventions.

The Ethical Mosaic of Biohacking

Biohacking, with its diverse practices and aspirations, is informed by a mosaic of ethical philosophies. Utilitarianism, deontology, and virtue ethics all play a role in shaping how biohackers approach self-improvement. What remains constant is the commitment to continuous ethical reflection and moral growth, ensuring that biohacking remains an ethical pursuit that benefits both individuals and society.

Ethical considerations are an integral part of the biohacking journey. Biohackers contend with complex dilemmas, seeking to balance personal ambition with responsibility, ensure safety and informed consent, and navigate the intricate moral landscape of self-improvement and human enhancement. By embracing ethical principles and reflecting on the impact of their actions, biohackers strive not only to be pioneers in self-optimization but also responsible stewards of the ethical dimensions of biohacking.

Other Chapter References

1. Caulfield, T. (2016). The Wild West of personalized medicine: Don't blame the consumers. Genome Medicine, 8(1), 57.

2. Grimaldi, K. A., et al. (2011). Ethical issues of bioinformatics. Bioinformatics, 27(6), 897–903.

3. Damschroder, L. J., et al. (2009). Fostering implementation of health services research findings into practice: A consolidated framework for advancing implementation science. Implementation Science, 4(1), 50.

4. Winstanley, E. L., et al. (2012). Design and use of a randomized crossover trial for the evaluation of complex interventions: The SHIFT study. Implementation Science, 7(1), 9.

5. Resnik, D. B. (2015). Informed consent in clinical research. In The Oxford Textbook of Clinical Research Ethics (pp. 693–702). Oxford University Press.

6. Emanuel, E. J., et al. (2008). What makes clinical research in developing countries ethical? The benchmarks of ethical research. Journal of Infectious Diseases, 198(5), 632-63.

7. Brown, R. (2011). Human universals. In Advances in Experimental Social Psychology (Vol. 44, pp. 1–51). Academic Press.

8. Kleinman, A., et al. (1978). Culture, illness, and care: Clinical lessons from anthropologic and cross-cultural research. The Annals of Internal Medicine, 88(2), 251–258.

9. Singer, P. (2011). Practical Ethics. Cambridge University Press.

10. Hursthouse, R. (2013). Virtue ethics. In E. N. Zalta (Ed.), The Stanford Encyclopedia of Philosophy (Summer 2013 Edition).

CHAPTER 12

THE FUTURE OF BIOHACKING

As the world of biohacking continues to evolve, the future holds exciting possibilities and some challenges. In this chapter, we explore the emerging trends and technologies that will undoubtedly shape the future of biohacking. This chapter discusses the democratization of biohacking, its potential impact on healthcare, and the relentless quest for human enhancement.

Emerging Trends and Technologies

Exploring Emerging Trends in Biohacking: The Future of Self-Optimization

Biohacking is a dynamic field that constantly adapts to new technologies and discoveries. By exploring emerging trends, we can gain insights into how these advancements are expanding the biohacking landscape.

The Rise of Artificial Intelligence (AI) in Biohacking

Artificial intelligence has revolutionized the field of biohacking by offering unparalleled capabilities in data analysis, pattern recognition, and predictive modeling.

- **Personalized Health Optimization:** AI-powered algorithms analyze vast datasets, enabling biohackers to personalize interventions with remarkable precision. From tailored nutrition plans to optimized sleep schedules, AI helps biohackers make data-driven decisions that align with their unique physiology and goals.

- **Health Predictions and Early Detection:** AI-driven health monitoring systems can predict and detect health issues before they become symptomatic. This early intervention empowers biohackers to address potential health challenges proactively.

Wearable and Implantable Technologies: The Future on Your Body

The integration of wearable devices and implantable technologies has brought biohacking closer to our daily lives than ever before.

- **Continuous Monitoring:** Wearable devices, from smartwatches to biosensors, provide real-time data on various physiological parameters. Implantable technologies offer even more granular insights, allowing biohackers to monitor internal processes with unprecedented accuracy.

- **Seamless Integration:** These technologies seamlessly integrate into biohackers' routines, providing constant feedback and facilitating rapid adjustments to optimize health and performance.

Innovative Biohacking Tools: From Lab to Home

Innovative tools and devices are being developed to empower biohackers in their self-optimization journeys.

- **DIY Labs:** Biohackers are increasingly building DIY labs at home, equipped with cutting-edge equipment for biochemical analysis, genetic testing, and experimentation. This democratizes access to scientific tools and accelerates bio-hacking research.

- **Biofeedback and Neurofeedback Devices:** Advanced biofeedback and neurofeedback devices offer real-time information on physiological and mental states. Biohackers use these tools to optimize meditation practices, manage stress, and enhance cognitive performance.

The Future of Biohacking: An Expansive Horizon

As we gaze into the future of biohacking, we see a horizon of possibilities. These emerging trends are reshaping the biohacking landscape, offering biohackers new avenues for self-improvement and a deeper understanding of their bodies and minds.

Expanding the Horizons of Biohacking: Beyond Physical Health

Biohackers are increasingly extending their focus beyond physical health and wellbeing by being cognizant of trends in neurohacking, cognitive enhancement, and the exploration of consciousness-altering techniques, such as nootropics and altered states of consciousness. In this way, biohacking converges with fields like neuroscience, psychology, and philosophy.

The Evolution of Biohacking: A Holistic Approach

Biohacking, once primarily focused on physical health, has evolved into a holistic endeavor that encompasses mental and cognitive aspects. Biohackers recognize that optimizing the mind is just as vital as optimizing the body.

Neurohacking: Unlocking the Brain's Potential

- *Cognitive Enhancement:* Neurohacking involves the deliberate manipulation of brain function to enhance cognition. This includes techniques such as brainwave entrainment, transcranial magnetic stimulation (TMS), and neurofeedback.

- *Nootropics:* Often referred to as "smart drugs," nootropics are substances that enhance cognitive function. Biohackers experiment with these compounds, striving to boost memory, focus, and creativity while closely monitoring their effects and safety.

Altered States of Consciousness: Exploring the Mind's Frontiers

- *Psychedelics:* Psychedelics have gained attention for their potential to induce profound altered states of consciousness. Biohackers engage in responsible and controlled psychedelic experiences to gain insights, address mental health concerns, and explore consciousness.

- *Meditation and Mindfulness:* Ancient practices like meditation and mindfulness are integral to biohacking. They offer pathways to altered states of consciousness and improved mental clarity, which biohackers incorporate into their routines.

The Interdisciplinary Nature of Biohacking

Biohacking's expansion into mental and cognitive optimization blurs the lines between the disciplines of neuroscience, psychology, and philosophy.

- *Neuroscience:* Biohackers draw on neuroscience research to inform their cognitive enhancement efforts. The field offers insights into brain plasticity, neurochemistry, and cognitive function.

- *Psychology:* Psychological principles underpin many biohacking techniques. Biohackers explore behavior modification, positive psychology, and cognitive-behavioral strategies to optimize mental wellbeing.

- *Philosophy:* The pursuit of altered states of consciousness and the exploration of human potential intersect with philosophical inquiries into the nature of self, consciousness, and reality.

The Multifaceted Nature of Biohacking

Biohacking's journey beyond physical health into neurohacking, cognitive enhancement, and altered states of consciousness reflects its multifaceted and interdisciplinary nature. Biohackers seek not only to optimize their bodies but also to unlock the full potential of their minds to embrace the complexity of human existence.

The Democratization of Biohacking

From Fringe to Mainstream

Biohacking is no longer confined to a niche community; it is moving into the mainstream. In fact, the democratization of biohacking is making self-optimization accessible to a broader audience through online communities, open-source resources, and affordable technologies in leveling the playing field.

- **Online Communities**: Online communities play a crucial role in democratizing biohacking. These communities provide a platform for enthusiasts, experts, and beginners to connect, share knowledge, and collaborate on various projects. They allow people from diverse backgrounds to come together, learn from one another, and discuss biohacking techniques and experiences.[456]

- **Open-Source Resources**: Open-source resources in software, hardware, and information are key to making biohacking accessible. Open-source projects provide access to tools and

---

[456] The Reddit subreddit r/Biohackers has over 60,000 subscribers and serves as a hub for discussions on DIY biology and biohacking techniques.

technologies that are often much more affordable than their proprietary counterparts. This enables individuals to experiment and innovate without significant financial barriers.[457]

- **Affordable Technologies**: Advances in technology have led to the development of affordable and accessible tools for biohacking. Devices like CRISPR gene-editing kits, lab equipment, and wearable sensors have become more affordable and user-friendly, allowing biohackers to conduct experiments and optimize their biology from the comfort of their homes.[458]

- **Educational Platforms**: Online platforms, courses, and tutorials have proliferated, providing education and guidance to those interested in biohacking. These resources enable individuals to gain knowledge and skills in biological sciences, bioinformatics, and DIY biology techniques.[459]

- **Bioethics and Safety Standards**: Alongside the democratization of biohacking, there is a growing emphasis on bioethics and safety standards. Online communities often promote responsible biohacking practices and encourage members to consider the ethical implications of their experiments.[460]

While the democratization of biohacking has expanded access to self-optimization, it is important to note that it also raises ethical, safety, and regulatory concerns. As more people engage in DIY

---

[457] The DIY Bio movement and organizations like the Open Insulin Project provide open-source protocols and tools for biohackers interested in creating insulin for diabetic patients.

[458] The CRISPR-Cas9 gene-editing technology has become more accessible with the availability of DIY CRISPR kits, such as the Odin Kit, which allows amateur biohackers to experiment with genetic modifications.

[459] Websites like DIYbio.org and Coursera offer courses and resources related to biohacking and DIY biology.

[460] Biohacker communities frequently discuss the importance of bioethics, and organizations like Biohack the Planet host events that include discussions on ethical considerations in biohacking.

biology, there is an increasing need for responsible practices, oversight, and dialogue between biohackers, regulators, and the wider scientific community to ensure that biohacking remains a force for positive change while minimizing potential risks.

Empowering Individuals

The future of biohacking is marked by empowerment in that biohacking tools and knowledge are empowering individuals to take control of their health and wellbeing. Today, self-quantification and personalized biohacking strategies are becoming the norm instead of the exception.

Biohacking tools and knowledge empower individuals to take greater control of their health and wellbeing in a remarkable way. In today's world, self-quantification and personalized biohacking strategies are rapidly becoming the norm, reshaping how we approach our health and lifestyles.

One of the primary drivers of this empowerment is easy access to health data. Wearable fitness trackers, smartwatches, and health monitoring apps have become ubiquitous, granting us instant access to a treasure trove of information about our bodies. From tracking our physical activity to monitoring our heart rate and even observing our sleep patterns, these tools empower us to maintain a continuous, real-time connection with our own physiology. Armed with this data, we can make well-informed decisions about our health and lifestyle choices.

- Continuous glucose monitors (CGMs) represent another breakthrough in the biohacking arena. These devices offer real-time tracking of blood glucose levels, offering vital insights for those managing conditions like diabetes. However, they are also used by biohackers interested in optimizing their diets and energy levels.

- DNA testing kits and services like 23andMe and AncestryDNA provide individuals with a deeper understanding of their genetic predispositions. Armed with this genetic information, people can tailor their health and wellness strategies to suit their unique genetic makeup.

- Personalized nutrition and fitness plans are now within reach, thanks to the combination of wearable data, genetic insights, and individual preferences. These customized plans ensure that our dietary and exercise choices align precisely with our goals and physiological needs.

- The use of nootropics (cognitive-enhancing substances) and supplements is widespread among biohackers to optimize mental performance and wellbeing. These enthusiasts openly share their experiences and recommendations within the biohacking community, fostering a culture of collaborative self-improvement.

Biohacking is not just about individual efforts, though; it thrives on the sense of community. Online biohacking communities and social networks have become hubs for knowledge sharing and support. Newcomers to the biohacking world can find a wealth of information, success stories, and strategies, making it easier than ever to join this empowering movement.

As we've previously discussed, biohacking is not merely confined to physical health; it extends to mental wellbeing. Wearables and apps that monitor stress levels, heart rate variability, and sleep quality enable individuals to manage their mental health more effectively. This holistic approach is an essential aspect of biohacking.

Biohackers are increasingly focusing on strategies to extend healthy lifespans. Interventions such as intermittent fasting, calorie restriction, and the use of anti-aging supplements and therapies are gaining popularity as people seek ways to age more gracefully and maintain their vitality.

Further, advanced bioinformatics tools and AI-driven health platforms are emerging to analyze large datasets and provide personalized health recommendations based on individual data. These tools are becoming indispensable in both healthcare and biohacking communities.

As awareness of biohacking grows through media coverage, books, podcasts, and documentaries, more people are embracing its potential benefits. This increased awareness is driving the widespread adoption of biohacking practices and strategies. However, while biohacking offers exciting opportunities for self-improvement, it's essential to approach these practices responsibly. Seeking professional guidance when necessary and considering ethical and safety implications is crucial. Integrating biohacking with conventional healthcare ensures a balanced approach to health and wellbeing.

The Potential Impact on Healthcare

Shaping the Future of Healthcare

Biohacking has the potential to transform the healthcare landscape in that its practices, data-driven approaches, and the integration of technology may lead to a more patient-centric, preventive, and personalized healthcare system. Biohackers may contribute to medical research and the development of innovative therapies.

- **Patient-Centric Healthcare**: Biohacking encourages individuals to actively manage their health by using data-driven tools and personalized strategies. This patient-centric approach puts individuals at the center of their healthcare, empowering them to make informed decisions and take proactive measures to maintain their wellbeing. Patients can track their vital signs, monitor chronic conditions, and make lifestyle adjustments, fostering a sense of ownership over their health.[461]

- **Preventive Medicine**: Data-driven biohacking practices emphasize the importance of early detection and prevention. By continuously monitoring health metrics and identifying trends, individuals can catch potential health issues in their early stages, allowing for timely interventions. This shift toward preventive medicine can lead to reduced healthcare costs and improved overall health outcomes.[462]

- **Personalized Treatment Plans**: Biohacking leverages data from wearable devices, genetic testing, and other sources to create highly personalized treatment plans. This tailoring of healthcare strategies ensures that interventions are not one-size-fits-all but instead align with an individual's unique physiology and genetic makeup. Personalized medicine is gaining traction, with treatments increasingly designed to target specific genetic markers or health profiles.[463]

- **Contributions to Medical Research**: Biohackers, who are often passionate and well-informed individuals, can contribute valuable data to medical research. By actively participating in research studies and sharing their health data, biohackers provide researchers with a wealth of information. Citizen science initiatives in biohacking can accelerate the pace of medical discovery.[464]

---

[461] Rathert et al. (2013). Patient-centered care and outcomes: A systematic review of the literature. Medical Care Research and Review.

[462] Green et al. (2002). Preventive medicine: The evolution of systems in health. Disease Management & Health Outcomes.

[463] Ginsburg, & McCarthy. (2001). Personalized medicine: A new medical and social challenge. Nature Reviews Genetics.

[464] Land-Zandstra et al. (2016). The rise of citizen science in health and biomedical research. American Journal of Bioethics.

- **Innovation in Therapies**: Biohackers, driven by their desire for self-improvement, often experiment with cutting-edge technologies and therapies. These experiments can lead to the discovery of novel treatments and interventions. For example, biohackers have explored the use of CRISPR gene editing and other emerging technologies, potentially contributing to the development of innovative therapies for various conditions.[465]

- **Data Sharing and Collaboration**: The biohacking community emphasizes data sharing and collaboration. Open-source platforms, forums, and communities allow biohackers to collectively analyze health data, share findings, and collaborate on research projects. This collaborative spirit can foster innovation and facilitate the rapid dissemination of knowledge.

- **Regulatory Considerations**: As biohacking practices gain prominence, regulatory bodies are adapting to ensure safety and ethical standards. Developing a regulatory framework that supports responsible biohacking while protecting public health is an ongoing process.[466]

Biohacking practices, data-driven approaches, and technology integration are paving the way for a healthcare system that is more patient-centric, preventive, and personalized. Biohackers, as active participants in this evolution, have the potential to enhance their own wellbeing and contribute to medical research and the development of innovative therapies, ushering in a new era of healthcare. This transformation holds the promise of better health outcomes and improved quality of life for individuals around the world.

---

[465] Barrangou, & Doudna. (2016). CRISPR-Cas9: A revolutionary tool for cancer modelling. Oncotarge.

[466] Bennett, M., & Chan (2018). Regulating the consumer internet of things: The UK and California experience. European Journal of Risk Regulation.

Ethical and Regulatory Challenges

The intersection of biohacking and healthcare presents ethical and regulatory challenges.

The rise of biohacking, driven by advances in technology and self-quantification, brings with it several critical issues related to privacy, data security, and the need for responsible oversight. While biohacking empowers individuals to take control of their health and wellbeing, it's crucial to strike a balance between individual autonomy and collective wellbeing in the biohacking community.

Privacy Concerns

- **Health Data Privacy**: With the extensive use of wearable devices and health monitoring apps, individuals generate vast amounts of personal health data. This data often includes sensitive information about their physical and mental health. Ensuring the privacy and security of this data is paramount. Unauthorized access or breaches can have serious consequences for individuals.[467]

- **Genetic Privacy**: Genetic testing, a common biohacking tool, raises concerns about the privacy of one's genetic information. This data not only reveals personal health insights but can also have implications for family members and future generations.

Data Security Issues

1. **Data Breaches**: Biohacking platforms and health-related apps are not immune to data breaches. The loss or theft of personal health data can lead to identity theft, blackmail, or unauthorized use of medical information.[468]

---

[467] Mittelstadt, & Floridi. (2016). Privacy in the age of medical big data. Nature Human Behaviour.

[468] Arora et al. (2017). The impact of data breaches on healthcare compliance: What can we learn from the literature? Journal of Healthcare Compliance.

2. **Ethical Hacking**: While ethical hacking can be a force for good, it also raises concerns about unauthorized access to medical devices or systems. Malicious biohackers could potentially compromise the security of medical technologies.

Responsible Oversight

1. **Ethical Considerations**: Biohackers need to consider the ethical implications of their actions, especially when experimenting with genetic modifications or unproven therapies. Ensuring that biohacking practices align with established ethical standards is crucial.

2. **Regulatory Frameworks**: The biohacking community, in collaboration with regulatory bodies, should work to develop responsible regulatory frameworks that ensure safety, protect privacy, and uphold ethical standards. Striking a balance between individual autonomy and collective wellbeing is challenging but necessary.[469]

3. **Public Awareness**: Raising public awareness about the potential risks and benefits of biohacking is essential. Informed individuals are more likely to make responsible choices and demand appropriate oversight.

Balancing Autonomy and Collective Wellbeing

1. **Informed Consent**: Individuals engaging in biohacking should be fully informed about the potential risks and consequences of their actions. Informed consent ensures that individuals understand the implications of their choices while respecting their autonomy.[470]

---

[469] Cwik, & Dowell. (2019). The ethics of biohacking: An inquiry into the right to perform genetic engineering on one's own body. Journal of Medical Ethics.

[470] Aldinger et al. (2014). Informed consent in human subjects research: A comparison of current international and South African guidelines. South African Journal of Bioethics and Law.

2. **Community Accountability**: The biohacking community itself can play a role in promoting responsible practices and setting ethical standards. Peer review and community guidelines can help ensure that biohacking remains a positive force for change.

3. **Collaboration with Healthcare Professionals**: Biohackers should collaborate with healthcare professionals and researchers to bridge the gap between self-experimentation and rigorous scientific investigation. This can lead to more responsible and evidence-based biohacking practices.

Balancing individual autonomy with collective wellbeing in the biohacking community is an ongoing challenge. While biohacking has the potential to empower individuals in their pursuit of health and self-improvement, it must be conducted responsibly, with due consideration for privacy, data security, and ethical considerations. Collaborative efforts between biohackers, regulatory bodies, and healthcare professionals are essential to ensure that biohacking continues to advance while safeguarding the interests of individuals and society at large.

Biohacking and the Quest for Human Enhancement

Pushing the Boundaries

Human enhancement has been a driving force in biohacking since its inception with a relentless quest for physical, cognitive, and emotional enhancement. This quest for physical, cognitive, and emotional enhancement has been a driving force in human history, reflecting our innate desire to improve ourselves. However, this pursuit raises profound ethical and philosophical debates surrounding the boundaries of human enhancement and the potential societal implications.

Physical Enhancement

- *Performance Enhancement*: Individuals seek physical enhancement to boost athletic performance, build strength, or enhance physical appearance. This often involves the use of supplements, drugs, or technologies to push the limits of human capability.

- *Aesthetic Enhancement*: Cosmetic procedures, such as plastic surgery and body modifications, allow individuals to alter their appearance according to their preferences. These enhancements blur the line between medical necessity and personal choice.

Cognitive Enhancement

- *Cognitive Boosters*: The use of nootropics, brain stimulation, and cognitive training techniques aims to enhance memory, concentration, and problem-solving abilities. These cognitive enhancers raise questions about fairness and the potential for cognitive inequality.

- *Neurotechnology*: Brain-computer interfaces (BCIs) and neuroimplants have the potential to enhance cognitive functions and even enable direct communication between humans and machines. These technologies challenge our understanding of consciousness and identity.

Emotional Enhancement

- *Mood-Altering Substances*: The use of drugs or substances to regulate emotions, reduce anxiety, or enhance positive feelings can have significant psychological and ethical implications. The balance between emotional wellbeing and chemical dependency is a key concern.

- *Neurofeedback and Mindfulness*: Techniques like neurofeedback and mindfulness meditation offer tools for emotional regulation and mental wellbeing. The ethical debate centers on the manipulation of emotions and the potential loss of authenticity.

Ethical and Philosophical Debates

- *Human Dignity*: Some argue that pursuing enhancements may undermine human dignity by suggesting that unenhanced individuals are somehow inferior. The question of whether enhancement violates our intrinsic value as humans is a central ethical concern.[471]

- *Fairness and Equity*: The availability of enhancements often depends on socioeconomic factors, raising questions about fairness and equity. If only the privileged can access enhancements, it may exacerbate existing inequalities.[472]

- *Safety and Long-Term Effects*: Many enhancements may have unknown long-term consequences. Ensuring the safety and efficacy of these interventions is a fundamental ethical challenge.[473]

- *Human Nature and Identity*: The pursuit of extreme enhancements can challenge our concepts of human nature and personal identity. How much change is too much, and at what point does one cease to be oneself?[474]

Societal Implications

- *Economic Productivity*: Enhanced individuals might contribute to economic productivity and innovation, but they could also

---

[471] Pellegrino, E. D., Schulman, A., & Thomas W. Merrill, T. W., eds. (2008). Human dignity and bioethics: Essays commissioned by the President's Council on Bioethics.

[472] Savulescu, J. (2005). Enhancement and equality. Philosophy & Public Affairs.

[473] Richter, K.W. (2011). Ethical aspects of genetic and psychopharmacological enhancement in children and adolescents. Ethics & Behavior.

[474] Chomsky, N, & Foucault, M. (2006). Human nature: Justice versus power: The Chomsky-Foucault Debate.

create divisions between enhanced and unenhanced populations, potentially leading to social unrest.

- *Healthcare Costs:* Widespread use of enhancements could strain healthcare systems, as they may be required to manage the health consequences of misuse or unforeseen side effects.

- *Privacy and Surveillance:* Neurotechnologies and data-driven enhancements may raise concerns about personal privacy and surveillance, especially if data about one's cognitive or emotional states becomes accessible to external parties.

- *Regulation and Governance:* Societies will need to develop regulatory frameworks to address the ethical and safety concerns associated with human enhancement. Striking a balance between personal freedom and collective responsibility is a complex task.

The relentless quest for physical, cognitive, and emotional enhancement represents a fundamental aspect of human nature. However, the ethical and philosophical debates surrounding the boundaries of human enhancement and the potential societal implications are complex. As we continue to push the boundaries of what is possible, it is essential to engage in thoughtful, informed, and inclusive discussions to shape the future of human enhancement in a way that aligns with our values and respects the dignity and wellbeing of all individuals.

The Transhumanist Vision

The potential for biohacking to play a pivotal role in the evolution of humanity and the ethical considerations associated with such endeavors is a reality. With a transhumanist vision of the future, we see that humans will merge with technology to transcend their current limitations.

Transhumanist Vision and Biohacking

- *Augmentation of Human Abilities*: Transhumanism envisions using technology to augment human abilities, including physical strength, intellectual capacity, and emotional well-being. Biohacking, with its focus on self-improvement and enhancement, aligns closely with this vision.

- *Integration with Technology*: Biohackers often experiment with technologies like brain-computer interfaces (BCIs), wearable devices, and genetic engineering to enhance their physical and cognitive functions. These technologies represent critical components of the transhumanist vision.

- *Lifespan Extension*: Transhumanists aim to extend human lifespans significantly. Biohacking strategies related to diet, exercise, and longevity research align with this goal, seeking to slow down the aging process and promote healthier, longer lives.

Ethical Considerations

- *Equity and Access*: As with many emerging technologies, there is concern that biohacking advancements may not be equally accessible to all. Ensuring equitable access to enhancement technologies is an ethical imperative to prevent the exacerbation of existing social inequalities.[475]

- *Human Identity*: The integration of technology into the human body raises questions about human identity. At what point does a person cease to be "human" and become something else? Ethical debates revolve around the potential loss of essential human qualities in the pursuit of enhancement.[476]

---

[475] Savulescu, J. (2005). Enhancement and equality. Philosophy & Public Affairs.
[476] Bostrom, N. (2003). The Transhumanist FAQ.

- *Safety and Risk Mitigation*: Biohacking experiments, particularly those involving unproven technologies or substances, can carry significant risks. Ensuring the safety of individuals who engage in biohacking is a paramount ethical concern.[477]

- *Regulatory Oversight*: Balancing individual autonomy with the need for responsible oversight is challenging. Establishing regulatory frameworks that safeguard public health while respecting personal freedom is an ongoing ethical debate.[478]

- *Societal Impact*: The widespread adoption of biohacking and transhumanist technologies can have profound societal implications, ranging from changes in social dynamics to potential conflicts over ethical values. Society must consider how these technologies will affect the collective wellbeing.[479]

Balancing Progress and Ethics

Achieving a balance between technological progress and ethical considerations is essential for the responsible development of biohacking and transhumanist technologies. This requires open dialogue, multidisciplinary collaborations, and the development of ethical frameworks that address issues such as equity, identity, safety, and regulation.

Ultimately, the future of biohacking and transhumanism hinges on our collective ability to navigate the complex ethical landscape while at the same time harnessing the potential for enhancement and transformation. As we continue to merge with technology to transcend our current limitations, it is incumbent upon us to ensure that

---

[477] Spittler et al. (2020). On the ethics of biohacking: Prevalence, motivations, and ethical justifications. BMC Medical Ethics.

[478] Müller, V. C. (2019). The ethics of enhancing intelligence: An assessment. Journal of Artificial Intelligence and Ethics.

[479] Luppicini, (2007). Societal and ethical implications of nanotechnology for the human body: An ethical perspective. Journal of Nanoparticle Research.

these advancements align with our values and respect the dignity and wellbeing of all individuals in an ever-evolving human-technological partnership.

As emerging trends and technologies shape the biohacking landscape, the democratization of biohacking empowers individuals, healthcare evolves, and the quest for human enhancement continues. Biohackers are at the forefront of this evolution, navigating ethical challenges and shaping a future where self-optimization is not only a possibility but a reality for all.

Other Chapter References

1. Hinton, G. E., & Salakhutdinov, R. R. (2006). Reducing the dimensionality of data with neural networks. Science, 313(5786), 504-507.

2. Han, S., et al. (2018). Wearable smart sensors integrated with cloud computing for effective real-time healthcare monitoring and early warning systems. Sensors, 18(3), 789.

3. Farah, M. J., et al. (2004). Neurocognitive enhancement: What can we do and what should we do? Nature Reviews Neuroscience, 5(5), 421-425.

4. Fadiman, J. (2011). The psychedelic explorer's guide: Safe, therapeutic, and sacred journeys. Inner Traditions/Bear & Co.

5. Reddit r/Biohackers: https://www.reddit.com/r/Biohackers/

6. Open Insulin Project: https://openinsulin.org/

7. The Odin CRISPR Kit: https://www.the-odin.com/diy-crispr-kit/

8. DIYbio.org: https://diybio.org/

9. Coursera - DIY Biology Courses: https://www.coursera.org/

10. Biohack the Planet: https://biohacktheplanet.com/

CONCLUSION

s you reach the final pages of this biohacking journey, pause, reflect, and contemplate the profound transformations you've already undergone. Your path through the chapters has led you to a deeper understanding of yourself, your body, and the limitless potential for self-improvement. To conclude, let's consider the importance of some of the key takeaways in this book.

1. Reflecting on Your Biohacking Journey

Take a moment to look back at the road you've traveled thus far. Recall the experiments you conducted, the knowledge you gained, and the challenges you faced. Reflect on the physical and mental changes you've experienced. Celebrate your successes and acknowledge the lessons learned from your setbacks. Remember that self-improvement is a journey, not a destination. The insights you've gathered along the way are invaluable, shaping not only your present but also your future.

2. Maintaining a Long-Term Biohacking Lifestyle

Biohacking is not a fleeting trend. Rather, it's a lifestyle that can continue to enrich your life in countless ways. Commit to maintaining the habits and practices you've cultivated. Consistency is key to long-term success. Stay engaged with the biohacking community, keep tracking your progress, and remain open to new discoveries and technologies that can further enhance your wellbeing. Both the journey of biohacking and the possibilities for self-improvement are limitless.

3. Inspiring Others to Join the Biohacking Revolution

To truly be the best version of ourselves, it's about more than personal growth. It's also about sharing knowledge and inspiring others to embark on their own biohacking adventures. As you continue to biohack your own life, become an inspiration for your friends, family, and community. Share your experiences, offer guidance, and foster a sense of curiosity and empowerment in those around you. By spreading the biohacking ethos, you contribute not only to a stronger version of yourself but to a healthier and more vibrant world.

4. Embracing the Power of Continuous Self-Improvement

Biohacking is not just a series of experiments or a collection of techniques; it's a philosophy that embraces the power of continuous self-improvement. The conclusion of one biohacking journey is merely the starting point for the next. Embrace the notion that you are a work in progress and your potential for growth is boundless. As you continue on your biohacking path, remember that the pursuit of optimal health and performance is a lifelong endeavor—one that promises a future filled with vitality, resilience, and the joy of self-discovery.

In closing, your biohacking journey is a testament to the human spirit's unyielding desire for growth and progress. As you turn the final page of this book, carry with you the knowledge that you are the author of your own biohacking story, and the possibilities for a healthier, happier, and more vibrant life are yours to explore and shape.

ACKNOWLEDGEMENTS

Writing this book has been a journey filled with countless moments of inspiration, perseverance, and growth. I owe immense gratitude to the following individuals and entities who have made this endeavor possible:

To my beloved husband, Alan, your endless encouragement, patience, and belief in me sustained me through every step of this process. Your unwavering support has been my greatest source of strength.

To my dear son, Tony, your understanding, brilliance, and patience during the moments when I was engrossed in my work were truly remarkable. Your love and understanding mean the world to me.

To my valued customers, your trust and support have been the driving force behind my passion for this work. Your feedback and enthusiasm have guided me towards creating something truly meaningful.

To my esteemed business partners, your collaboration, insights, and shared vision have enriched this project beyond measure. Together, we have overcome challenges and celebrated successes, forging a bond that I deeply cherish.

To Hasmark Publishing International, thank you for believing in my vision and providing the platform to bring it to life. Your professionalism and dedication to excellence have been invaluable throughout this journey.

To my editors, Deanna and Sigrid, your expertise, guidance, and attention to detail have elevated this manuscript to new heights. Your contributions have shaped this book in ways I could not have achieved alone.

To my parents, your unwavering belief in me and your encouragement to always strive for the highest level have been my guiding light. Your faith in my abilities has fueled my determination, and I am forever grateful for your love and support.

To all others who have played a part, whether big or small, in bringing this book to fruition, I extend my heartfelt thanks. Your contributions have left an indelible mark on this journey, and for that, I am profoundly grateful.

With deepest appreciation,
Grazyna Pajunen, Ph. D.

ABOUT THE AUTHOR

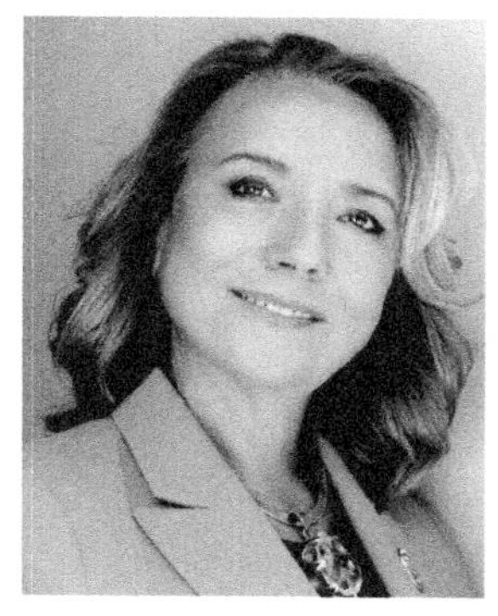

Born in Warsaw, Poland, Dr. Grazyna Pajunen is a dynamic blend of academia and innovation. She holds a Master's degree in Solid State Electronics from the Technical University in Warsaw and a Ph.D. in automatic control systems from the Helsinki University of Technology, Finland.

Drawn to the US for her impressive expertise, Dr. Pajunen has enriched students for over 25 years with her teachings at institutions like Florida Atlantic University and UCLA. Beyond her academic contributions, her in-depth research in her field has resulted in over 50 refereed publications. As a testament to her innovative spirit, she also collaborated with industry giants, earning her 15 US patents with Motorola.

Despite her illustrious academic and professional journey, an inner calling prompted Dr. Pajunen to pivot her focus. Captivated by the potential of holistic health and reversing the aging process, she transformed her passion into credentials by becoming a board-certified functional nutritionist.

Today, she co-leads a successful anti-aging venture alongside her son, a certified health coach. Together, they offer a beacon of hope to those seeking to decelerate the aging process. Their holistic approach aims to help clients avoid invasive measures, emphasizing a life free from discomfort and wrinkles without relying on medications, injections, or surgeries. For Dr. Pajunen and her son, their mission is more than just a profession—it's a passion, with a genuine commitment to transforming lives through health and wellness.

FOR FURTHER RESOURCES PLEASE VISIT:

http://AgeReversingSecret.com
http://BeDiscomfortFree.com
https://Effectivecollagen.com

SOCIAL MEDIA NETWORK/HANDLES:

https://Linkedin.com/in/gpajunen
https://YouTube.com/@grazynapajunen

email: info@effectivecollagen.com

BOOK A 15-MINUTE CONSULTATION:
https://meetme.so/bewell

AVAILABLE NOW ON AMAZON

Made in the USA
Las Vegas, NV
14 February 2025

18118025R00157